CONQUER CROHN'S

Josh MacDonald

Copyright © 2020 Josh MacDonald

All rights reserved.

ISBN: 9781700577726

For the waitresses who don't roll their eyes when I tell them I have dietary restrictions.

ii

CONTENTS

Acknowledgments   i

My Story   1

You Have a Disease   5

Part I: Lifestyle   7

Part II: Medication   13

Part III: Diet   30

Part IV: Training   47

ACKNOWLEDGMENTS

To my doctor, Dr. Khursheed Jeejeebhoy and his caring nurse, my aunt Tracey.

To my trainers, Ryan and Lloyd. I'd be lost in the gym without your teachings. I now know what it means to train hard.

To the man who encouraged me to start training and to write this book, my friend Don. Get jacked or die tryin'.

To those who participate in my IBD surveys and polls. The data I've gathered for this book, my videos and my blog will help thousands of people.

To everyone who helped with the contents of this book. Everett and Chase for the cover help. Abbey for the long nutrition chats.

To whoever created the app Flipp. You've helped me save a lot of money on chicken and egg whites.

MY STORY

I woke up from an afternoon nap in my 1950s-styled dorm room and vomited directly into my trash can. I didn't have a stomachache. I hadn't been drinking. I was exhausted, from what I thought were my 8am lectures. I wasn't necessarily studious, but I'd never skip lectures to sleep in.

I was 18 when I started college at Queen's University in Kingston, Ontario. I was living in residence. During the start of the semester, I always thought the cafeteria food wasn't that bad. This gradually changed.

I would grab a tray, grab a couple plates of food, 4 glasses of milk and sit down with a group of friends at a large table. I'd take one bite of food and claim I'm not hungry, even though I hadn't eaten for 6 hours. Some of my friends were getting sick of the food at the time and would pick through their food. We all brushed my lack of appetite off as a product of the cafeteria food quality.

We started eating off campus. Same thing. I wasn't hungry. A hot slice of pizza, or a burger at a local burger joint – nothing. I wasn't hungry.

Fortunately, the school year ended, and it was time to head home for the summer and work at the family business. Dad wanted me to do physical labor work, mainly because that's what he did growing up for some reason.

The cooking at home was much better, but my symptoms were not. I'd start work at 8am and finish at 5pm, with a half hour lunch break. I'd carry large, heavy blocks used to support 25,000 pounds boats while they were pulled out of winter storage for customers to access for the upcoming summer season.

I recall one of my lowest points before diagnosis. It would have been a Friday evening. I was at a local bar with my family and another family. I ordered a delicious pasta dish, and when it came out of the kitchen, it was heavily steaming. The smell of the food alone was enough to trigger my nausea to the point I had to go outside for fresh air, before ever taking a bite. I sat down on a cement parking stop to maintain consciousness.

Something was definitely wrong.

Later I drove home, and my family followed as soon as they were done their meals. I spent the evening dry heaving over the toilet, on the cold tile floor. My 105-pound body, shivering on the floor with every attempt to empty, my already empty stomach. It was awful.

I was always skinny and tall. I measure 6'2" (and would probably be taller without Crohn's slowing growth) and never surpassed 130 pounds in my life. I quit hockey at 13 because I was just too small for the body contact. How I miss it.

I ended up sleeping from that Friday night into Sunday morning. I didn't wake up for Saturday. Sunday, we decided to head to the local ER where they gave me fluids and I was able to go home. I started visiting different doctors, and running blood work, searching for a diagnosis. I was given some pill, which I think was placebo, it didn't help.

Canada's slow healthcare system eventually diagnosed me with Crohn's disease around my 19th birthday. Prednisone was the drug that pulled me out of that rut like magic. An amazing drug with nasty side effects. But that drug saves lives so I'm thankful for it.

Fast forward a few years, Crohn's was under control through

medication and strict diet, it was time for surgery to remove the scared parts of my bowel. Fortunately, I only had 15cm removed.

I remember waking up after my surgery, trying to stand up but projectile vomiting constantly. I've already been fasting for 2 days, so the fact I was still losing fluid was alarming. More alarming, my blood cell count was lower than that of a newborn baby.

Before this surgery began, I was informed that there was an 8% chance I needed a blood transfusion, and I was in that 8%. More so, the blood transfusions weren't helping. One transfusion, then another, then part way through another I remember the doctor on my floor calling for an emergency surgery.

It was Saturday night, so they had to call the surgeons in. The porter was taking too long to come get me, so the doctor pushed my bed, kicking doors open with her feet, rushing me into surgery like something out of a Grey's Anatomy episode. The nurse, a kind lady, told me she was praying for me as she passed me off to the surgeons. My parents were crying, as I think they were more scared of the idea of death than I was. I was pretty calm. If it was my time to go, then it was my time to go. Sometimes your name is called earlier than expected.

I was brought into the cold surgery room, now with about 7 different hoses (IVs and such) hooked to my body. There were 4 or so doctors around me. I was on heavy meds at this point, but I still remember calmly asking them to please save me and then I was put to sleep. I remember waking up the next day to crying people, the person in the bed next to me didn't make it.

Throughout the following pages, I'm going to walk you through how I was able to go from this state of 105 pounds, to add over 50 pounds of nearly entirely lean muscle mass to create a healthy, strong, respectable and attractive physique.

A short disclaimer. I am not a doctor. I am not a health professional of any kind. The information I provide is based on being proactive with my disease. I want more than anything in this world for all of us to get better and I want to bring you along for the ride.

YOU HAVE A DISEASE. ACT LIKE IT.

This isn't really applicable to most of you because you're currently reading a book on your disease. Majority of those with IBD, are not. Some are posting photos of fast food in Facebook groups because they "were craving it" meanwhile they've been trying to escape a month-long flare. Some are constantly drinking alcohol and wondering when the next magic pill is going to be invented to heal their gut and allow them to live like a normal, binge-drinking, fast-food-eating, unactive person. Okay, this is an exaggeration, but there are many people out there who come to mind when I read the description above. Please, do not act like them.

Do as your doctor says. Talk to other intelligent people with the disease. Go on Google News and search "Crohn's disease" to read the latest. Watch YouTube videos on it. Just be proactive and don't expect a cure to be handed on a silver plate, even though we all deserve one at this point.

"Some never get control of it, and those ones die." said my nurse, who is also my aunt. This is an acknowledgement you have to make, and it might help you power through this book, apply my teachings and take your disease more seriously.

It's important to be proactive with your disease while you still have lots of your bowel left to work with. Eating meals through a gastric feeding tube or through intravenous feeding is not part of an enjoyable life. Eventually the Crohn's may continue to spread, and surgeons will run out of parts to remove. With that said, I want to quote something I read in a group from a patient by the name of Lisa Stowe.

"I am diagnosed with end stage Crohn's. There are no longer treatment options available for me. I was told at the time that it is incredibly rare to get that diagnosis. I had heard of a couple of others with the diagnosis, but they've passed on since.

A bit of background on my case. Thirteen surgeries over a eleven-year period. I can't have oral medications at all. Can't do biologics due to cancer history. I have a ton of unique side effects that play into my issues. Liver damage, hair and tooth loss, psoriatic arthritis, lack of absorption issues. My hospital team is at a loss now. I just keep moving forward."

Lastly, I want you to embrace that it's difficult. Use the pain to find strength. If you win this battle, it is rewarding. It's something to be proud of. Being a heathy individual is rare in North America, let alone healthy with a disease. Seriously. Go to the mall and look around. It's full of sloppy people who are out of shape, and statistically speaking, they have nothing wrong with them - as in no disease. For many of them, laziness and comfort has got them to the spot they're in. We aren't going to be like that. Having a healthy body with Crohn's disease really is something exceptional to be proud of. When you internalize that and achieve such, you will become extremely happy, proud and confident.

It's not all sunshine and rainbows though. People won't understand why you're so proud of your progress. People won't understand your newfound obsession – and yes, getting healthy with Crohn's disease will become an obsession. You'll be told things like "there's more to life than the gym" from people who never seen the inner walls of a gym. They just won't get it. Your discipline might even startle some because it shines weakness on them. They don't know what it's like to eat the same meals every week and be happy doing it. They won't understand the discipline it takes to go a year straight without training less than 4 times a week and letting absolutely nothing get in the way of it. They are different than us and that's okay, but don't let their insecure comments or lack of care for their health get you off your path. Leave them be. Let your friend circle shift to people aligned with your goals. Stay focused and reap the rewards of your labor. I am so excited for you.

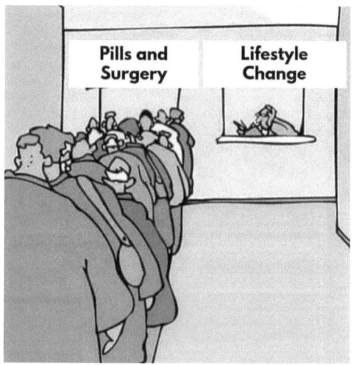

Modern society's mindset.

PART I: LIFESTYLE

I'm going to skip the boring *what is Crohn's* introduction and get right to a practical guide of navigating Crohn's disease and ulcerative colitis, the other form of IBD (irritable bowel disease). Identifying triggers is going to be the most important step to getting better. Lifestyle changes alone won't put your disease in remission but if you don't know what elements of your lifestyle trigger you to feel awful, it will be hard to avoid it. If you're recently diagnosed, you're likely in a constant flare and anything and everything has the same, painful effect. It's up to medication like prednisone to pull you out of this rut, then it's your turn to have an attempt at taking over with a proper lifestyle.

With someone in remission like myself, it usually takes more than one trigger to activate a flare. A few missteps in my diet won't cause much of a reaction, but maybe if I ate fast food for dinner, drank a bunch of alcohol late that night, got no sleep and woke up to some sort of news that causes stress, that could cause a flare. If I ate a good dinner, had some junk food for a snack, drank alcohol and then got a solid peaceful rest, I'd probably be fine if I only did it sparingly.

Often to stimulate a flare with a patient in remission, all the holes of the swiss cheese need to align. Similar to what I was taught in pilot school about airplane crashes – multiple things need to go wrong before everything as a whole goes south. A flare can last a day, or it can last years. Mine generally last a day or two at this stage thankfully.

After surveying several people with IDB, stress is the most common trigger and voted to be the number one trigger in more than 95% of patients. Stress can be caused in an infinite amount of ways, but it's been said nothing will create more pain in your life than financial stress. It can also be from school or work. Relationships can also cause stress. If you're friends with people who cause stress, you can usually rid of them, but if you're married to them, or they are your offspring, this is obviously different.

Most colleges seem to have some sort of disability or accessibility division where they take your doctor's documentation of your disease and offer you resources. After I transferred to the University of Toronto (to be closer to my family) I was offered many services like note-taking and private testing facilities. I was allowed several hours' worth of bathroom breaks with stopped time during my exams and tests.

Work options change based on your field. I am self-employed and my staff work remotely, so both them and I have flexibility with the hours we work, breaks, etc. If you're also in the tech space, many employers offer great perks to attract talent.

Outside of the tech space, there are other opportunities to find jobs with flexibility. Electricians are often on-call 24 hours and can take selective jobs. Substitute teachers also take workdays as they wish. I have a friend, she's an actuary, and she starts her workday when wants as long as she puts her hours in and gets her work done. If you are self-employed, for example if you owned a boutique spa, you could easily move clients around if you were in a flare.

Trainers, journalists (or any writer for that matter… PR, copywriter, bloggers, content marketers, email marketers, translators), house keepers, rideshare drivers, dispatchers and call center representatives are all jobs with high flexibility. The list is quite extensive, and it gets bigger with your creativity.

Building on business hours, waking up early is another

trigger for myself. I sleep 9 to 10 hours normally and when I'm training heavily, I sleep 10 to 12. Sleeping longer helps with recovery, more on this later.

Going to bed earlier is an obvious solution, but if I had to get up for 6am, I would be in bed by 8pm. That's a little ridiculous. Imagine being on a date and the other person tells you they have to be home by 7:30pm. Weird. At my young age, going to bed at 11pm and getting up at 9am is much easier to mesh with society. At an older age, in a marriage with young kids for example, obviously going to bed earlier and waking up earlier is more common.

Speaking of marriage, partner selection is extremely important. If you're not married currently, please pay attention. The number of stories I read about marriage conflict around this disease is alarming. Marriage is the number one most important decision you will make in your life, with or without the disease. Finding the right partner and being the right partner is incredibly important for everyone.

To avoid conflict, many have suggested others to either never get married or marry someone who also have the disease. Both fine options, but rash.

Surely, living alone with Crohn's as your grow old could prove difficult. It's difficult living as an elder, even without disease. The people considering avoiding marriage are usually so set on the idea that discussing it further won't change their decision.

Marrying someone with Crohn's is also a great option, but your candidate pool is going to be smaller. You'll likely have to use internet dating and be open to traveling long distances to meet.

Personally, I am not a marriage expert. However, I spend a bit too much time reading books, some of those have been psychology books on relationships, which has led me to not follow either of the above options. The topic of relationships causes lots of disagreement but I'm going to touch on them anyways as it is important.

You really need to be good at analyzing people and

testing them, and there needs to be solid attraction from the start to build upon. The topic of attraction alone could be a 10-book series and there are already books on it, so covering it wouldn't make sense.

Often, I think to myself when on a date, is there anything I could tell this woman to scare her off? Although not my intention on my first few dates, I'm able to place my finger on the idea of whether this is going to be a short-term thing or something that has the possibility of going the length.

Short-term is great when you're 24. I generally don't tell new women I have Crohn's and I advise you to adopt a similar practice when dating – just hide it the best you can. In the odd chance they might ask where I got my belly scars and I banter a sarcastic fib while I maintain focus on opening the next bottle of wine, but generally they're too shy and respectful to ask. When attraction builds after several dates and we are considering enter a relationship, that's a suitable time for me to break the news - and if I've analyzed my partner correctly, nothing will change what we already have going. For those with low self-esteem, you will get hurt if you reveal it and don't get a follow-up date. Determine if the person is worthwhile first.

Obviously the higher she is attracted to me (physically, emotionally, mentally, etc.), the more she'll deal with me and my disease. If she is head-over-heels for me, and if I can maintain that level of attraction (and eventually love) for decades to come (a difficult feat) then surely, having a disease won't change much.

People often get into relationships because one is just as desperate as the other, when there's no real attraction there other than biological needs. This isn't enough to carry a relationship, especially if one has a disease. Ideally if I'm looking for a girlfriend, I'll go on a dozen dates with women who I know like me. 10 of them will want a second date and half of them I'll want a second date with. Probably 3 would turn out to be high quality, looking to please me at any opportunity, meaning the attraction is really high. This is what a relationship needs. These 3 women are the women who would eventually discover I have Crohn's disease. From those 3, I use intuition over the course of 10-20 dates deduce to the one to pursue a relationship with.

When you're that selective, you end up finding amazing partners who will give you nothing but support for your battle.

A girl that relates to my disease on an emotional level is going to understand me better than one who's never experienced such. As an example, from my past, an ex-girlfriend of mine had been close to cancer, a more common disease, via her father and her grandfather.

I was sick, and my physical appearance was subpar thanks to extreme weight loss, but it didn't change anything. She was very attracted to me and cared much for me throughout our relationship. In fact, she cared more about my health and disease than I did. She was a fitness influencer, so she was very passionate about me getting into the gym. I had this belief that I couldn't put on weight until surgery, so I eventually quit going to the gym the first time around, and focused on my business, which was doing very well at the time.

That relationship caused stress for me at time, which caused flares. The stress was partly as a result of mistakes on my part and the rest as a result of her instinct to pray on the fact I was inexperienced. I had never been in a relationship until then, so entering my first relationship as a sophomore with a sorority girl, far more attractive and social than me and nearly 3 years older… was a learning experience to say the least. I'm thankful for the learning experience but being single after that certainly caused less stress for me and my disease. I believe that's why so many IBD patients believe single is the key – because they haven't experienced an optimal partner.

School, job and partner selection are the primary choices you need to optimize to lower stress in your life, but it doesn't stop there. Depending on when you were diagnosed, you'll be faced with new opportunities and different paths your life can take going forward. Having kids is a big one.

Like normal people, you should consider if you and your partner can afford to support a child and give them a quality life. I read years ago that the average kid costs $250,000 to raise and it's probably a lot more now. I was probably a solid multiple of that number to raise if I had to guess.

What's different for people with Crohn's is you need to make the judgement whether you can still afford a child, if you were off work permanently due to Crohn's. Can your partner support the whole family? Do you have enough money saved instead? Will your parents help out? Can you collect disability?

Please, please, please do not have children if you can't give them, and yourself, a quality of life you all deserve.

In addition to the financial aspect of children, it is of general agreement by health professionals that your Crohn's should not be active during conception[1].

In a study in The American Journal of Gastroenterology, they analyzed childbirths from mothers with inactive Crohn's disease. 24.6% of births were small for gestational age (SGA) births in the Crohn's group, compared with only 1.5% in the group without.

Although it's evident that Crohn's can affect the birth of your offspring, most people with IDB have no family history of it, meaning it likely won't be passed down.

On the off chance that one of your children get IBD, you will at least be able to efficiently aid in them in their battle and you'll understand how important your support is. Not everyone with the disease has the blessing of supportive parents. My parents do good more than they don't, but I got to where I am because of me. I had limited support from my parents. They don't always understand how important good nutrition and physical activity is, along with the attention this disease demands and that leads to family conflict. I'm not saying this to seek sympathy from my readers - I'm saying this to tell you that it happens even to people who may look successful from the outside looking in. It's best to acknowledge that these people are family and you can't trade them for someone else. Move forward and realize people like yourself can still accomplish great things without support. Try to stay focused on your goals and let no

---

[1] Moser, M A, et al. "Crohn's Disease, Pregnancy, and Birth Weight." The American Journal of Gastroenterology, U.S. National Library of Medicine, Apr. 2000, www.ncbi.nlm.nih.gov/pubmed/10763954.

one pull you from that and if you have loved ones that actively support you, cherish it.

In general, when it comes to unsupportive people in your life, focus on isolating yourself, and if it's family, moving out and distancing yourself early would be a good first step to focus on. This will lower stress and improve the overall quality of your life.

By identifying your triggers and crafting a lifestyle around your Crohn's disease with careful consideration of the concerns listed in this chapter, you can start building yourself a high-quality life immediately.

PART 2: MEDICATION

Your first goal with medication should be to get off it. Most of these medications have serious side effects. If you're anything like me, you get a bit uncomfortable when you see your medication on a TV commercial and the voiceover starts listing the possible side effect, with the last side effect on the list always being death.

Medication is a temporary fix. There is no medication that is a permanent fix. Patients often switch from one drug to the next when it stops working. Seriously sad stories occur when you start running out of drugs to try. That will push your life into the deep end.

"Hard times create strong men. Strong men create good times. Good times create weak men. And, weak men create hard times." is an old quote that applies nicely here.

Do not slack because times are good. Good times will bring out comfort in you, and comfort results in not paying attention to triggers. I don't think I need to walk you through where this is going.

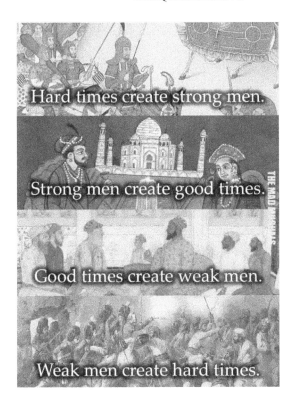

Medications change and differ based on insurance coverage which depends on where you live, among other things, so me recommending one isn't going to help you. However, I will recommend some common medications to research in alphabetical order.

Your doctor will provide recommendations and like anyone else giving information, it could be helpful or not. Do consider that some doctors receive commission for referring patients to certain drugs.

Adalimumab (Humira)
Humira, classified as a tumor necrosis factor blocker, is the drug I am on at the time of writing this. I take it with methotrexate. After the loading dose, I take 1 self-injected pen every 2 weeks.

It is pretty painful, although there's a new Citrate-free version out in certain countries that doesn't cause as much pain. At the time of writing this, it's available in the USA but Canada has yet to approve it. Humira has been able to put 4 out of 5 Crohn's patients into remission[2]. It has been recognized as "the world's best-selling drug"[3] and the national average drug acquisition cost (NADAC) is $2,521 per pen[4] and most patients take two pens per month.

Azathioprine (Azasan, Imuran)
An oral medication, Azathioprine has been around for decades with many success stories. It's typically used to prevent organ rejection after a transplant and can also treat arthritis. This drug is an immunosuppressant which works by lowering your body's immune system.

Certolizumab pegol (Cimzia)
Certolizumab pegol is the first biologic on the list which primarily lists Crohn's disease as one of the indications. The FDA approved Cimzia for the treatment of Crohn's disease in 2008. With a half-life of 11 days, your doctor will advise shots to be taken as frequent as Humira shots (which has a half-life of 20 days), or sooner.

Esomeprazole (Nexium)
Esomeprazole is a medication used to treat acid reflux and GERD (gastroesophageal reflux disease). Some doctors also prescribe it to prevent ulcers. It is often taken orally, twice a day.

Hyoscyamine (Levbid)

---

[2] Sandborn, J, et al. "Adalimumab for Maintenance Treatment of Crohn's Disease: Results of the CLASSIC II Trial." Gut, BMJ Publishing Group, 1 Sept. 2007, gut.bmj.com/content/56/9/1232.short.

[3] Mukherjee, Sy. "Protect at All Costs: How the Maker of the World's Bestselling Drug Keeps Prices Sky-High." Fortune, Fortune, 15 Jan. 2020, fortune.com/longform/abbvie-humira-drug-costs-innovation/.

[4] "NADAC as of 2019-02-27." Centers for Medicare and Medicaid Services, data.medicaid.gov/Drug-Pricing-and-Payment/NADAC-as-of-2019-02-27/s7c9-pfa6.

Extracted from plants, Hyoscyamine is the only natural medication on the list. With a wide variety of uses, Hyoscyamine is known to lessen symptoms in the lower abdominal area, which would include bladder diseases, ulcers, pancreatitis, in addition to irritable bowel syndrome among other things. This orally administered drug will help with your cramps.

Infliximab (Remicade)
Infliximab is another popular medication used to treat a similar list of autoimmune diseases similar to Humira. It is administered through intravenous, often every 8 weeks. Medically in use since the 90s, Infliximab can cost Americans between $5000 to $16000 if they do not have insurance.[5]

Mercaptopurine or 6-MP (Purixan)
Mercaptopurine is a medication used to treat both cancers and different forms of irritable bowel syndromes. It is often used with methotrexate. Orally administered, this drug is much more affordable than most on the list. Like any other oral, liver toxicity is a known side effect so routine blood tests are to be expected.

Mesalamine (Lialda, Apriso, Mezavant or Pentasa)
Used to treat both mild to moderate cases of Crohn's disease and ulcerative colitis, Mesalamine is another orally administered drug, costing slightly more than 6-MP. Although more uncommon than some of the others on the list, Mesalamine has its fair share of success stories online and had to be included in the list. It can also be taken rectally.

Methotrexate
In addition to Humira, I take Methotrexate. Although it can be taken orally, I take it by subcutaneous injection. You can also take it via intravenous or intramuscular injections. Available as a

---

[5] "How Much Does a Remicade Infusion Cost?" What Is the Price How Much Does a Remicade Infusion Cost Comments, www.howmuchisit.org/remicade-infusion-cost/.

generic medication, methotrexate is likely the cheapest medication on the list. It's been in use for over 60 years, and World Health Organization's List of Essential Medicines lists the drug as one of the safest and most effective medicines needed in a health system.

Pantoprazole (Protonix)
Similar to Esomeprazole, Pantoprazole is taken to treat ulcers and acid reflux. It is also administered by mouth.

Prednisone
A corticosteroid, prednisone is used to suppress the immune system. It's affordable and is extremely effective. A major side effect is weight gain. Given it's administered orally and is metabolized by the liver, it can cause liver damage so while extremely effect with IBD, is only a short-term solution.

Pulmicort (Entocort, Budesonide)
Pulmicort is a corticosteroid, like Prednisone, and used to treat mild-to-moderate IBD. It can also only be taken for a limited time. Three months is a common treatment length. Dosages are often front loaded then tapered as quitting immediately is dangerous. Unlike Prednisone, it's available in many forms of administration such as orally and rectally but also as a nasal spray and inhaler.

Sucralfate (Carafate)
Similar to Pantoprazole and others, Sucralfate is used to treat ulcers, to prevent ulcers, treat GERD and reduce stomach inflammation. It can be administered both orally and rectally.

Tofacitinib (Xeljanz)
Similar to Humira and Remicade, Tofacitinib or better known as the brand name Xeljanz is used to treat different types of arthritis and ulcerative colitis. It is administered orally via tablets and has a very short half-life of 3 hours which means dosing would need to be frequent.

Ustekinumab (Stelara)

Ustekinumab is a monoclonal antibody used to treat psoriasis, Crohn's disease and ulcerative colitis. The half-life is roughly 3 weeks and can be administered by either by subcutaneous injection, or by infusion.

Vedolizumab (Entyvio)

Vedolizumab is another monoclonal antibody used to treat Crohn's disease and ulcerative colitis. Unlike many others on this list, this drug was developed primarily for IBD.

I surveyed about 50 people with Crohn's and ulcerative colitis and to little surprise, these were the common answers. Some I've never heard of, so I was happy to research and include those. If Humira loses its effectiveness, Stelara is at the top of my list to try next. I have an acquaintance who is on it, and he gives self-injections only every 8 weeks, which is appealing. 6 or 7 injections per year? That would be amazing.

With that all that being said, I think Western doctors are too quick to prescribe a drug that costs $70,000 per year like Humira when it's clear there are numerous studies out there for cheaper alternative medication – and I'm not even a doctor. Remember, the goal of big pharma is money, not your health.

I want to share some studies I've found around alternative medication. Based on my research, the categories that I think are worth discussing are hormones, peptides and cannabis. Before I present the studies, I should warn you to not do anything illegal. Abide by the laws of your country. If I thought this information was useless to those with Crohn's disease, I wouldn't include it. What you do with this information is up to you.

First, let's talk about hormones. There is plenty of research linking higher testosterone in men with dramatically lower Crohn's disease activity suggesting men with lower testosterone may be at risk of moderate to severe instances rather than mild. The studies we will discuss are mainly testing benefits in men, as there hasn't been much research for treating Crohn's disease in

CONQUER CROHN'S

women with hormones. While women have testosterone, their levels are 15-18x less than a typical male, on average.

For those unfamiliar with the traditional uses of exogenous hormones, many men in their 40s and beyond are on hormone replacement therapy (HRT) from their doctors as their natural productions have slowed. Hormones like testosterone keep men young and motivated. It boosts energy levels, lean muscle mass and sex drive. It improves sleep, mood and cognition. It decreases LDL (bad cholesterol) and body fat.

When it comes to IBD, hormones can aid in both lowering your CDAI (Crohn's disease activity index) and increase bodyweight.

After reading the studies that follow, the benefits will sound unbelievable, but there are side effects and risks that your doctor will be able to walk you through. You can then analyze your quality of life presently with the stage of your disease and determine if the risks associated are worth improving that. The answer is different for each person.

There are five exogenous hormones I'm going to discuss that are readily available from doctors in many countries. The first is testosterone. This is the most widely used. You probably know someone who is privately on testosterone replacement therapy (TRT) from their doctor, as it is widespread in North America. Older men can easily get a testosterone prescription from their doctor if their testosterone is low. It's mainly an injectable but also available as an oral, and it's been proven to improve the clinical course of Crohn's disease[6].

---

[6] Nasser, Mahmoud, et al. "Testosterone Therapy in Men with Crohn's Disease Improves the Clinical Course of the Disease: Data from Long-Term Observational Registry Study." Hormone Molecular Biology and Clinical Investigation, De Gruyter, 12 June 2015, www.degruyter.com/view/j/hmbci.2015.22.issue-3/hmbci-2015-0014/hmbci-2015-0014.xml.

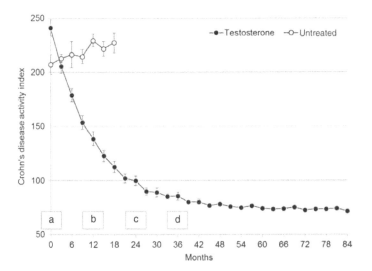

Figure 1: Effect of testosterone administration on CDAI in 92 men receiving testosterone compared to 14 men receiving no testosterone (mean±SEM). b vs. a, p=0.001; c vs. b, p=0.02; d vs. c, p<0.05.

This 2015 study by Nasser et al explains "In total, 92 men received parenteral testosterone undecanoate 1000 mg/12 weeks for up to 7 years. Fourteen men opted not to receive testosterone and served as a comparison group. In men receiving testosterone, the Crohn's Disease Activity Index declined from 239.36±36.96 to 71.67±3.26 at 84 months (p<0.0001 vs. baseline). C-reactive protein levels decreased from 12.89±8.64 to 1.78±1.37 mg/L at 84 months (p<0.0001 vs. baseline). Leukocyte count decreased from 11.93±2.85 to 6.21±1.01×109/L (p<0.0001 at 84 months vs. baseline). No changes were observed in the comparison group. There were no significant side effects of testosterone." This study makes it clear that testosterone has a direct link in men to their Crohn's Disease Activity Index (CDAI).

A 2010 study ran a similar test in men aged 45-67. The study explains "Upon normalization of serum T (testosterone), there was a significant decline of CDAI (from 243±19 to 89±9), CRP levels from 22.7±8.1 to 6.9±2.9 mg/dL, and white blood cell count. Hemoglobin/hematocrit increased significantly. Upon normalization of plasma T, the CDAI and CRP levels decreased in hypogonadal patients with CD. The mechanism of this improvement could be through immunosuppressive effects of T, reducing chronic inflammation of the intestinal wall in CD."[7]

Testosterone levels can be improved naturally and don't necessarily require exogenous administration. One of the major benefits that come with strength training is increased testosterone. In 2006, Andrada et al. from the University of Extremadura, had 20 male volunteers follow a 4-week strength training routine. The individuals had no training experience, and the following chart shows the increase in their testosterone after following the program for 4 weeks.

	Values before the programme		Values after the programme	
	Before the session (A)	After the session (B)	Before the session (C)	After the session (D)
Testosterone	38.73 ± 17.54	33.00 ± 15.64	53.00 ± 45.55	29.00 ± 19.73
Epitestosterone	13.27 ± 6.37	11.73 ± 6.36	21.64 ± 14.45	12.18 ± 6.36
Androstenedione	3.09 ± 1.6	3.00 ± 1.5	4.9 ± 3.1	2.9 ± 1.1
Dehydroepiandrosterone (DHEA)	13.72 ± 8.2	11.0 ± 6.32	17.54 ± 14.5	9.9 ± 6.54
Androsterone	1,736 ± 850	1,527 ± 790	2,596 ± 1,990	1,468 ± 1,250
Etiocholanolone	1,420 ± 974	1,249 ± 750	2,124 ± 1,740	1,202 ± 780

---

[7] Haider, Ahmad, et al. "Administration of Testosterone to Elderly Hypogonadal Men with Crohn's Disease Improves Their Crohn's Disease Activity Index: a Pilot Study." Hormone Molecular Biology and Clinical Investigation, Walter De Gruyter, 8 June 2015, www.degruyter.com/view/j/hmbci.2010.2.issue-3/hmbci.2010.033/hmbci.2010.033.xml.

Additionally, sleep duration is linked to higher testosterone. I used to limit my hours of sleep because I thought it had an overall benefit in my daily productivity. Little did I know, it was killing my testosterone.

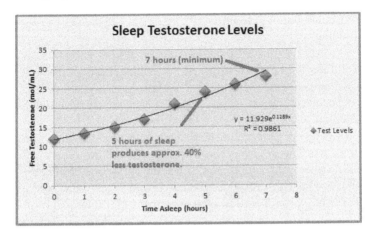

In addition to strength training and getting sufficient rest, eat a clean diet containing sufficient protein, fat and carbs. Minimize stress and get some sun.

Men who are low in vitamin D tend to also be low in testosterone and consequently, men who have sufficient vitamin D tend to have dramatically higher testosterone levels. Individuals should take 2000-3000 IU per day.[8]

Magnesium, zinc and boron are also staple vitamins proven to increase testosterone that every man should take, with Crohn's disease or not. Often, I find over-the-counter daily vitamins don't include zinc, so I recommend spending the extra money and finding a good multivitamin. Optimum Nutrition makes a comprehensive vitamin that costs a bit more but is well worth it. They also make a women's version too with proper dosing. For those with a larger multivitamin budget, Rootine

---

[8] Wehr, E., Pilz, S., Boehm, B.O., März, W. and Obermayer-Pietsch, B. (2010), Association of vitamin D status with serum androgen levels in men. Clinical Endocrinology, 73: 243-248. https://doi.org/10.1111/j.1365-2265.2009.03777.x

offers a customized micronutrient solution that you can tailor based on tests and other data points.

Ashwagandha is a supplement known for combating stress, but multiple human trails show it also increases testosterone. It becomes especially effective when used in conjunction with resistance training. Reportedly, the effective daily dose is 500-1000mg.

Shilajit, also called mineral pitch, is a sticky substance that develops as a result of plant matter breaking down is commonly used in ayurvedic medicine and has shown in two human trials to positively impact testosterone levels. The effective dose is 200mg daily.[9][10]

Creatine is a common supplement in the bodybuilding world and numerous studies show its positive effect on testosterone. Some forms of creatine can cause some digestive side effects so those of us with Crohn's disease may need to test a few types to find what works best. The common types of creatine are creatine monohydrate, buffered creatine (Kre-Alkalyn), creatine hydrochloride (HCL), and creatine nitrate.

D-aspartic acid, mucuna pruriens, tongkat ali, forskolin and royal jelly all have some evidence of increasing testosterone but none of them have as much concrete evidence as the initial supplements we discussed.

Many overhyped supplements tend to negligibly increase testosterone or not work at all. These supplements include Tribulus terrestris, horny goat weed, maca, saw palmetto, stinging nettle and velvet antler.

Supplements, particularly those aimed at hormonal balance, often require a few months to demonstrate noticeable effects. Obtaining blood work, both pre- and post-intervention, is a reliable method to gauge their impact on testosterone levels. In

---

[9] Biswas TK, Pandit S, Mondal S, Biswas SK, Jana U, Ghosh T, Tripathi PC, Debnath PK, Auddy RG, Auddy B. Clinical evaluation of spermatogenic activity of processed Shilajit in oligospermia. Andrologia. 2010 Feb;42(1):48-56. doi: 10.1111/j.1439-0272.2009.00956.x. PMID: 20078516.

[10] Pandit S, Biswas S, Jana U, De RK, Mukhopadhyay SC, Biswas TK. Clinical evaluation of purified Shilajit on testosterone levels in healthy volunteers. Andrologia. 2016 Jun;48(5):570-5. doi: 10.1111/and.12482. Epub 2015 Sep 22. PMID: 26395129.

the USA, you can use privatemdlabs.com to order a requisition form online. In the UK, you can try medichecks.com and bluehorizonmedicals.co.uk. In Canada, most doctors won't write a blood requisition for testosterone checks for someone under the age of 40 but you can go to a walk in and say you're showing signs of low T and that you're going to try to boost your testosterone with supplements and would like to monitor your levels. You can also use an online doctor to get a requisition, specifically getmaple.ca, or cross the border to the US.

Consistent monitoring is key to understanding the effectiveness of any treatment regimen. Adjustments based on testosterone level changes can significantly impact the management of Crohn's Disease. This strategy underscores the importance of empirical evidence in guiding treatment choices, rather than solely relying on subjective symptoms.

When initial interventions do not yield the expected results, considering alternative options becomes necessary. This decision should be informed by a thorough evaluation of potential benefits and risks. Such a calculated approach is critical in chronic conditions management, where the goal is to find the most effective, personalized strategy for each individual.

It is evident across these two studies alone that testosterone significantly improves an individual's CDAI. In the next studies, we will look at additional benefits, like weight gain.

Nandrolone decanoate acts on the androgen receptor to elevate testosterone levels. Its medical use extends to promoting muscle growth, enhancing appetite, boosting red blood cell production, and improving bone density, making it a versatile injectable therapy. Its efficacy in these areas opens up discussions on its broader applications, particularly in chronic conditions where these benefits could be crucial.

In a study highlighted by Anthony M. Kasich, nandrolone phenpropionate's intramuscular injections were analyzed for their effect on 48 underweight patients suffering from various gastrointestinal disorders. The weekly administration resulted in significant weight gain, with particularly remarkable outcomes in ulcerative colitis cases. Notably, the treatment exhibited no hepatotoxicity or signs of fluid retention, suggesting its safety profile alongside its therapeutic benefits.[11]

Although research into nandrolone's direct impact on disease progression is limited, its potential benefits for patients suffering from severe undernutrition due to Crohn's Disease are significant. Crohn's Disease's adverse effects on growth, bone density, and puberty highlight the need for effective treatments. Nandrolone's capacity to address these issues presents a compelling case for its consideration in comprehensive disease management plans.

Oxandrolone, marketed under the brand name Anavar, stands out as an orally administered medication approved in the Western world for medical use, particularly for inducing weight gain. Its mechanism, akin to that of nandrolone, facilitates an increase in testosterone levels, offering a unique advantage in therapeutic settings where oral administration is preferred.

Research involving oxandrolone in the treatment of growth and puberty delays in teenage boys has shown promising results. A notable study by Stanhope et al. revealed that administration of oxandrolone significantly accelerated growth velocity compared to a placebo, highlighting its potential as an effective intervention for related developmental delays.[12]

The administration of these hormonal therapies requires careful management due to their potential to suppress natural testosterone production. Gradual cessation and possibly the introduction of other medications are necessary to restore endogenous hormone levels safely. Moreover, the process of aromatization can lead to elevated estrogen levels, necessitating additional considerations in treatment planning. A study from

---

[11] KASICH, A M. "CLINICAL EVALUATION OF NANDROLONE PHENPROPIONATE IN PATIENTS WITH GASTROINTESTINAL DISEASE." The American Journal of Gastroenterology, U.S. National Library of Medicine, Dec. 1963, www.ncbi.nlm.nih.gov/pubmed/14099447.

[12] Buchanan, et al. "Double Blind Placebo Controlled Trial of Low Dose Oxandrolone in the Treatment of Boys with Constitutional Delay of Growth and Puberty." Archives of Disease in Childhood, BMJ Publishing Group Ltd, 1 May 1988, adc.bmj.com/content/63/5/501.abstract.

CONQUER CROHN'S

2019 further elucidates the complexity of hormonal interactions, underscoring the importance of comprehensive monitoring and management in hormonal therapy.[13]

The last hormone I want to mention is growth hormone (GH). There have been studies that show growth hormone could be a beneficial treatment for those with Crohn's disease but the problem with all these hormone options I've offered is that is doctor generally won't prescribe a generic drug, because we all know there's no money in that. Their jobs revolve around patents forcing patients to pay for expensive drugs.

This is the only drug I've presented to my doctor and he says he's only done it once for a patient and that one patient had side effects so he's hesitant to encourage me to try it. Additionally, Canada won't let him prescribe such drug for Crohn's disease, so his patients that are interested in such he sends to the United States. If this did work, my doctor risks me dropping my existing prescriptions. I once read a disclaimer on the receptionist's desk about how certain doctors are compensated by third parties for the work they do – basically hinting at the fact that he may or may not get money for putting his patients on specific drugs.

The study I want to share with you consists of 37 adults with moderate-to-severe active Crohn's disease. They were divided into two groups – a placebo group and a GH group. The GH group injected GH every day and followed a high protein diet, similar to the amounts I recommended earlier.

Conducted in 2000, Slonim et al explain "At base line, the mean ($\pm$SD) score on the Crohn's Disease Activity Index was somewhat higher among the 19 patients in the growth hormone group than among the 18 patients in the placebo group (287 ± 134 vs. 213 ± 120, P=0.09). Three patients in the placebo group withdrew before their first follow-up visit and were not included in the data analysis. At four months, the Crohn's Disease Activity Index score had decreased by a mean of 143 ± 144 points in the growth hormone group, as compared

---

[13] "Five Anabolic Steroids in the Treatment of Inflammatory Bowel Disease." Journal of Gastroenterology Research, Scholarly Pages, 7 Sept. 2019, scholars.direct/Articles/gastroenterology/jgr-3-019.php?jid=gastroenterology.

CONQUER CROHN'S

with a decrease of 19±63 points in the placebo group (P=0.004). Side effects in the growth hormone group included edema (in 10 patients) and headache (in 5) and usually resolved within the first month of treatment." [14]

In conclusion, "our preliminary study suggests that growth hormone may be a beneficial treatment for patients with Crohn's disease."

It's now clear that there is some benefit to using hormones to treat Crohn's disease. While they may take more work on behalf of the patient and have risks associated with them, any serious patient should read these studies (the links at in the footnotes of each page) and bring them to their doctor if they're interested in them. If your doctor isn't open minded to stemming from traditional options, ask another doctor.

In the contemporary discourse on hormonal therapies, the conversation extends to include SARMs (Selective Androgen Receptor Modulators) and peptides. Despite their chemical differences, they often appear together in discussions due to their potential therapeutic applications. SARMs, in particular, represent a newer class of compounds, with most having emerged in the last two decades, marking them as areas of keen interest for future research and development.

A primary advantage of SARMs lies in their selectivity, aiming to minimize side effects associated with traditional testosterone therapy by offering tailored responses. For instance, RAD-140, a SARM under early clinical investigation, boasts a remarkable androgenic to anabolic ratio of 1:90. This specificity suggests potential for more targeted and efficacious treatments, prompting a reevaluation of current therapeutic approaches.

The anabolic properties of a drug enhance anabolism, or cell growth, facilitating muscle development. This process involves increased protein synthesis and appetite, alongside muscle enlargement, contributing to strength gains. The distinction

---

[14] Slonim, A E, et al. "A Preliminary Study of Growth Hormone Therapy for Crohn's Disease." The New England Journal of Medicine, U.S. National Library of Medicine, 1 June 2000, www.ncbi.nlm.nih.gov/pubmed/10833209.

between anabolic and androgenic effects is critical in understanding the therapeutic potential of these compounds.

Androgenic effects, on the other hand, relate to virilization side effects, including acne and hair thinning. While not guaranteed, these risks are pertinent to treatments like testosterone, which exhibits an androgenic to anabolic ratio of 1:1. Consequently, lower dosages are often prescribed to balance therapeutic benefits against potential adverse effects.

One notable advantage of SARMs, including Ostarine, LGD-4033, and RAD-140, is their oral administration, offering a contrast to the injectable, patch, or gel forms of testosterone. This method of intake, however, prompts considerations regarding liver health, with the full extent of impact still under study. Despite the lack of prescription availability, these compounds have garnered interest for their potential to provide muscle-building benefits akin to anabolic hormones but with a profile of milder side effects, as perceived by the public.

Although SARMs lack extensive research concerning Crohn's disease, their emerging profile warrants mention for future considerations. Given testosterone's significant impact on CDAI, it raises the question of whether SARMs could present similar therapeutic advantages with an improved safety profile.

MK677, though not classified as a SARM, frequently appears in related discussions. As a growth hormone secretagogue, it stimulates increased GH production, offering a cost-effective alternative to direct growth hormone treatments. Its role in enhancing GH and IGF-1 levels facilitates lean muscle gain without fat accumulation, also improving hunger and REM sleep patterns. These effects contribute to more effective calorie consumption and recovery, highlighting its potential in broader therapeutic applications.

The aforementioned study indicates that GH administration can positively affect CDAI, underscoring the therapeutic potential of hormone modulation. However, it is crucial to acknowledge the possibility of side effects, including receptor overstimulation leading to adverse mental health outcomes. This highlights the importance of a balanced approach in therapy, weighing benefits against potential risks.

It is anticipated that the coming decade will bring an expansion of research on SARMs, particularly in exploring their effects on inflammatory bowel diseases (IBD). This growing body of knowledge will be crucial in determining their viability as part of IBD management strategies.

Beyond hormones, SARMs, and secretagogues, peptides represent another avenue of treatment that has garnered both anecdotal and preliminary scientific support for their role in Crohn's disease management. Composed of short sequences of amino acids—the fundamental components of proteins—peptides are more readily absorbed by the body, suggesting their potential for therapeutic efficacy.

The peptide I want to draw attention to specifically is BPC-157. It's a sequence of amino acids derived from human gastric juice. Gastric juice is dangerous when in contact with the throat and can cause significant inflammation. BPC-157 is known for its healing properties. It's taken by numerous athletes with tendon or muscle injuries. The regenerative effects of BPC-157 have been experienced by thousands of people across the web.

Although widely used recreationally by humans who have taken their injury healing upon themselves, BPC-157 has yet to begin human trials in treatment of IBD. It was shown to have promising effects in rats but never pursued further.[15]

If you're not interested in talking to your doctors about any of these advancements, but want to try something new, do consider clinical trials. Rochester, MN, La Crosse, WI, Jacksonville, FL, and Scottsdale/Phoenix, AZ all have active clinical trials at The Mayo Clinic for Crohn's disease. At the time

---

[15] Vuksic T, Zoricic I, Brcic L, Sever M, Klicek R, Radic B, Cesarec V, Berkopic L, Keller N, Blagaic AB, Kokic N, Jelic I, Geber J, Anic T, Seiwerth S, Sikiric P. Stable gastric pentadecapeptide BPC 157 in trials for inflammatory bowel disease (PL-10, PLD-116, PL14736, Pliva, Croatia) heals ileoileal anastomosis in the rat. Surg Today. 2007;37(9):768-77. doi: 10.1007/s00595-006-3498-9. Epub 2007 Aug 27. PMID: 17713731.

of writing, there are currently 34 listed on their website.[16]

With all this talk of Western medication, I can't go any further without talking about cannabis. I created both a blog post and a YouTube video on the topic if you haven't seen those yet. Search "Conquer Crohn's" on YouTube to see the help videos I've created or visit ConquerCrohns.ca to see all of my blog posts.

Sativa is generally used in medicinal purposes over indica. For those new to the topic, sativa and indica are the two types of cannabis. Sativa is known to reduce stress and increase mental capacities like creativity and focus. Indica is known for its relaxation properties and generally feels stronger than sativa.

For those with IBD, sativa is mainly used for its medicinal benefits. There are also hybrids, where you can get some benefits of both types.

Cannabis contains multiple compounds called cannabinoids. The main cannabinoids discussed are known by their acronyms as CBD and THC. In successful studies, people mainly smoked joints with high THC content. CBD, in the recent years, has been a topic of hype.

Since I was unable to find any academic studies on the success of CBD while treating IBD, I'm not recommending it. However, there's nothing wrong with picking a strain of cannabis that contains both THC and CBD. There are many strains, with different ratios to choose from.

The final thing I need to cover with cannabis is the fact that cannabis is known to have a placebo effect. People consume cannabis and expect good things, because there's plenty of hype around it. People who consume placebo cannabis have found their placebo cannabis helped them with their IBD. Because of this, I do encourage you to be honest with yourself and consider it may not have helped as much as you think it did.

Cannabis isn't the only natural remedy that's shown to be promising in the treatment of Crohn's disease. Grape seed extract has been promising in one study with mice. Interleukin

---

[16] https://www.mayo.edu/research/clinical-trials/

10 (IL-10) is an anti-inflammatory cytokine which has been linked to IBD. Both ulcerative colitis and Crohn's disease are associated with defective IL-10 signaling resulting in deficiencies. A 2014 study found that grape seed extract suppresses inflammation in IL-10-deficient mice.[17]

Uncaria tomentosa is a vine commonly known as cat's claw and is another agent widely known for it anti-inflammatory effects. A study done on rats concludes Cat's claw protects cells against oxidative stress and negated the activation of NF-$\varkappa$B (a protein complex that controls transcription of cytokine production).[18] Anecdotal of one user says they started at 500mg of cat's claw during a flare and would work up to 4500mg to stop a flare.

Wormwood (artemisia absinthium)[19] also has some dated studies showing benefits in treatment of Crohn's disease. Additionally, helminths (that would be parasitic worms)[20] and fecal transplants have been tested and, in some cases, shown to be effective in treatment.

---

[17] Yang G, Wang H, Kang Y, Zhu MJ. Grape seed extract improves epithelial structure and suppresses inflammation in ileum of IL-10-deficient mice. Food Funct. 2014 Oct;5(10):2558-63. doi: 10.1039/c4fo00451e. Epub 2014 Aug 19. PMID: 25137131.

[18] Sandoval-Chacón, , Thompson, , Zhang, , Liu, , Mannick, , Sadowska-Krowicka, , Charbonnet, , Clark, and Miller, (1998), Antiinflammatory actions of cat's claw: the role of NF-$\varkappa$B. Alimentary Pharmacology & Therapeutics, 12: 1279-1289. https://doi.org/10.1046/j.1365-2036.1998.00424.x

[19] Omer B, Krebs S, Omer H, Noor TO. Steroid-sparing effect of wormwood (Artemisia absinthium) in Crohn's disease: a double-blind placebo-controlled study. Phytomedicine. 2007 Feb;14(2-3):87-95. doi: 10.1016/j.phymed.2007.01.001. Epub 2007 Jan 19. PMID: 17240130.

[20] Radford-Smith, G L. "Will worms really cure Crohn's disease?." Gut vol. 54,1 (2005): 6-8. doi:10.1136/gut.2004.044917

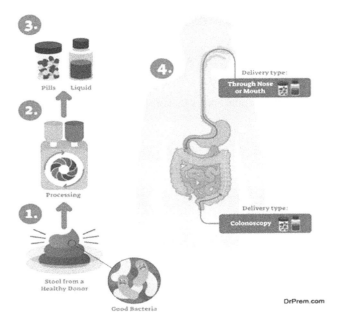

Unfortunately, much of these studies are not overly promising or haven't been studied for one reason or another. Like kimchi, kombucha and kefir, some of these less-studied supplements probably can't put you in remission alone but sometimes when your disease takes a turn for the worst, you'll try anything for a chance at having a better day.

PART III: DIET

Can diet solve IBD alone - a question that is commonly debated, usually in quite heated discussions online. The only way I could see diet alone treating Crohn's or ulcerative colitis would be if you caught the disease early and figured out your diet immediately. You could potentially stop the inflammation before it grew too much – but that's all speculation and the chance you catch the disease early is almost zero.

Crohn's disease is widely considered an autoimmune disease, not a digestive disease. It is a disease that affects the gastrointestinal (GI) tract, however. Given our food goes through the GI tract, it's best we take precautions with what we put through it to avoid additional issues.

To answer the opening question, it's well established that there are no cures for this disease, but there are treatments and measures we can take to stop progression of it. I believe, anecdotally, poor diet can cause pain by increasing inflammation. A good diet won't necessarily cure you or make you symptom-free, but it will help lower inflammation.

There are many people who claim diet alone has kept them in remission for decades, so there are very few reasons to not take diet seriously.

For starters, safe foods within your diet can be found using an elimination diet which is the process of removing foods from your diet that you suspect may be causing issues. This is tricky. You might order a hamburger from a restaurant. A couple hours later, you're sick to your stomach. In a hamburger, there's the bun, the red meat, maybe some hot peppers – which are all possible culprits. You ordered it without cheese because you already concluded dairy gives you pain.

What else is on your hamburger? Ketchup, mustard, maybe some pickles. You had a hot dog for lunch with almost no issues, so it can't be the bun. You had a steak last night safely, so it can't be the red meat. You always eat hot peppers with no pain. What gives?

You might walk away from this now and say "it had to be the bun" because now with consideration, you've convinced yourself the hot dog from earlier did give you some mild temporary pain. That may have been related to breakfast though, but you forgot about that possibility. Don't worry, I do too, and these are the problems you run into with an elimination diet.

What's missing in this consideration is the fact that most restaurants load up their buns with butter or the fact that the bun at lunch was white and this one was whole wheat. Sure, whole wheat is considered to be "healthier" because of the micronutrients (which can be obtained from a good multivitamin) but it's harder to break down whole wheat bread than white bread. Whole wheat bread is also higher in fiber and some doctors suggest a low-fiber diet to treat IBD. Let's assume it was the butter, however. Sometimes the button is on the inside so it's not visible. Many people don't know this. You might. Pizza crusts are the same way. The last time I ate at a Pizza Hut was probably 15 years ago because they're known for putting butter on everything.

Butter is the ultimate cheat. Nearly any dish, even if it's dog food, can taste better with butter. If you're a bad cook, you can always just call it a day and put butter on it. Cheese works too. This is why it's so common for butter or cheese to be on many dishes in a restaurant.

So now I've showed you how elimination diet can easily put you on the wrong path, you will hopefully be more thoughtful and thorough when reflecting on each meal you eat.

When running an elimination diet, it's helpful to look at lists of foods that are known to cause issues with IBD. I have some on my blog, but you can also Google for them but sometimes the writers for blogs that appear on Google have little to no experience in what they're talking about. On my blog I regularly add foods that I believe are safe for the majority and unsafe for the majority.

Everyone's diet is different and what works for one might not work for another, but there are usually similarities. Often anything with insoluble fiber should be avoided: corn, seeds, nuts, raw leafy greens, raw thick skinned veg, etc.

If you read on a forum that a food that is safe for 90% or more people, and you believe it causes pain, I suggest you consider retesting the food. With such a small number of people claiming the food hurts them, I often encourage others (in the least offensive way possible) to consider the inaccuracy of the testing they did to reach that conclusion. I use this strategy to find new foods to consider adding to my diet.

Besides elimination, you can visit a naturopath. This is a tender subject for some, but I've found their testing beneficial. The problem with naturopaths, like any industry, is you have people who are legitimately helpful and those who scam. It's up to you to read reviews and talk to friends to find reputable professionals.

These clinics can run a blood test on you, usually a finger prick, which will provide a multi-page report on food intolerances. Before doing one, you want to try to eat a balanced diet, including some of everything. Eat dairy, eggs, all the meats, fish, fruits, vegetables, etc. If you exclude certain foods from your diet before the test, their potency may be downplayed in the results.

The test is a few hundred dollars, so not many people do it, but some will jump at any opportunity to potentially improve the course of their disease by even a fraction. Of those

I know who have done this test, they swear by it. I base a lot of my diet off this, but I'm always challenging and retesting results. I stay proactive.

Other types of diets include low residue, low fiber, paleo and many others. I can't speak for all of them.

Personally, my diet, while a combination of the above, falls closest to a paleo diet. The easiest way someone described a paleo diet to me is if it flies, walks, swims or grows in/from the ground, I'll eat it. Basically, one ingredient foods. No breads. No dairy. Over the years since adapted that diet, I've found exceptions like if it's white bread, I will eat it or if its acidic like pineapple, I won't eat it. It gets complicated when you realize white bread is acidic, which is why there's no diet carved in stone for IBD patients. It comes down to regular testing to see what is responding best with your gut. If you want to be safe you could just stick to water but what kind of life would that be?

"so what CAN you eat?"

me:

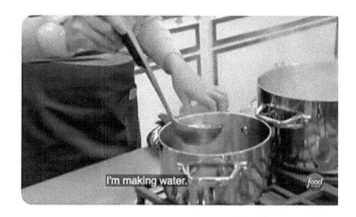

There are all sorts of diets out there, and many studies contradict another. For example, one study took 64 patients with Crohn's disease. Half of them were treated with a fiber-rich, unrefined-carbohydrate diet and the other half had no dietary instruction. The group with a monitored diet spent a total of 111 days in the hospital compared to 533 of the group with no dietary instruction.[21]

How can this be possible if most doctors recommend a low fiber diet? I'm not in a position to answer that. However, I am in a position to tell you that diets differ for all of us. Perhaps the fiber-rich diet, although maybe not optimal, unintentionally

---

[21] Heaton, K W, et al. "Treatment of Crohn's Disease with an Unrefined-Carbohydrate, Fibre-Rich Diet." The BMJ, British Medical Journal Publishing Group, 29 Sept. 1979, www.bmj.com/content/2/6193/764.abstract.

avoided more well-known problem foods such as dairy or red meat by focusing on fiber-rich foods which may have been the real cause of success in the experimental group. The control group ate everything, which may or may not have had fiber, but they had a higher chance of eating foods with low fiber like dairy and red meat which have zero fiber.

Plant-based diets also appear frequently in online discussions as they are a hot topic in both nutrition and social justice. When vegans and vegetarians push a certain diet for social justice reasons, they back it up by additional facts not related to the core reason. This is what confuses people. For example, a plant-based diet is often pushed for environmental benefits. Activists persuade such a diet by adding additional (and often true) claims. A plant-based diet will be better for IBD patients than an uncontrolled diet because it cuts out things like fast food and processed food, but it also cuts out foods which are safe with most IDB patients like chicken or fish. Do you know what's also healthier than a normal diet? A diet containing both meat and plants that still avoids fast food and processed food. You don't have to quit meat entirely, you can just focus on lean meats like chicken, fish and turkey.

As for a less enjoyable diet, an elemental diet has been found to be "as effective as corticosteroids in the treatment of previously untreated Crohn's disease"[22] with corticosteroids being medication like prednisone. An elemental diet is usually a powder blend that can be mixed and drank, or in more severe cases administered through a gastric feeding tube or intravenous. This diet is usually composed of amino acids, fats, sugars, vitamins, and minerals. I've never done it. I've never needed to after I discovered its effectiveness. It lacks protein but if you are in a flare, or don't need high protein because you're not exercising (which you should be), then this would be worthwhile to try as this research has been proven effective over numerous studies, including studies that only tested a 'half

---

[22] Payne-James, J J, et al. "Initial Response and Subsequent Course of Crohn's Disease Treated with Elemental Diet or Prednisolone." Gut, BMJ Publishing Group, 1 Sept. 1993, gut.bmj.com/content/34/9/1198.abstract.

CONQUER CROHN'S

elemental diet'.[23]

One study suggested some popular problem foods. These foods were "wheat, corn, dairy products, citrus fruits, tea and coffee"[24]. Another claimed, "Food intolerances discovered were predominantly to cereals, dairy products, and yeast."[25]

Spicy foods and alcohol are also generally accepted to make symptoms worse. I occasionally drink socially, and you can too if you can keep it to an occasion.

Although my diet will be different from yours, I'm going to walk you through a typical daily diet for me. I have five meals – some big and others small.

Meal one is anything along the lines of eggs, home fries, cereal or Cream of Rice, with a glass of apple juice (not from concentrate). Orange juice is fine too, but I'll only choose that if the grocery store has the low acid variant in stock. Again, no added sugar when it comes to picking juices. This meal will usually focus on giving me energy from both simple and complex carbohydrates. I'm starting to add in a protein shake in the mornings with this first meal, so I hit two macros off the bat. More on macros later.

Meal two is usually after I train – late morning. This is a muffin, a banana and raw egg whites. Egg whites can be cooked, but I can drink more of them raw, and quicker. Given I eat five meals per day, I don't have time to just sit around, cooking and eating. You could also do another shake here if you rather something with flavor.

If you want to try it, don't make your own egg whites. You buy the egg whites in cartons next to eggs in your grocery store. These are pasteurized and put into cartons. Do not eat

---

[23] Takagi, S., et al. "Effectiveness of an 'Half Elemental Diet' as Maintenance Therapy for Crohn's Disease: a Randomized-Controlled Trial." Wiley Online Library, John Wiley & Sons, Ltd, 9 Oct. 2006, onlinelibrary.wiley.com/doi/full/10.1111/j.1365-2036.2006.03120.x.

[24] Levi, A J. "Diet in the Management of Crohn's Disease." Gut, U.S. National Library of Medicine, Oct. 1985, www.ncbi.nlm.nih.gov/pmc/articles/PMC1432936/?page=3.

[25] Riordan, A.M., et al. "Treatment of Active Crohn's Disease by Exclusion Diet: East Anglian Multicentre Controlled Trial." The Lancet, Elsevier, 21 Sept. 2003, www.sciencedirect.com/science/article/pii/0140673693921219.

raw unpasteurized egg whites. If you want help with flavor, mix it with Nesquik. It will taste great with that. If you have the money, try MuscleEgg.

Meal three is my first big meal. This is either chicken, turkey or fish for protein, and sweet potatoes, quinoa or rice for carbs. Sometimes I'll give the option of pasta. Veggies are usually a good idea for overall health as they have micronutrients, but they don't aid in gaining weight because they're low in calories. I often boil my chicken, then shred and season with taco seasoning but you can cook it however you like. I often make many days' worth at once. Meal four is the same as this meal, just 3 hours later.

Last meal is meal five, which I often drink a shake. The shake can contain whatever you'd like but generally mine contains:

- 50g of protein from egg whites or protein powder
- 1 banana
- 1 cup of strawberries (5 or 6)
- 1 cup of oats
- 2-3 tablespoons of avocado oil (good fats with no taste)
- ½ cup of oat milk
- Water if you added protein powder
- Vanilla extract if your protein powder tastes bad

I blend this together and it measures about 1.25 liters, which is just over ¼ of a gallon, and contains nearly 1000 clean calories. I drink this at my desk, while I finish work before bed. It takes 45 minutes to sip on, or about half that if I focused on it. It's not a mojito, but it tastes great.

Speaking of mojitos, I rarely drink. I live in Canada, so I hibernate in my igloo in the winter. However, in the summer as a young male, it's hard to not drink here and there – more so when I'm single and in the mood to party. If you are on medication that can cause liver toxicity, you must be careful. Drinking lots of water, steadily, can help with the liver. I don't mean a few glasses a day when you remember, but a lot of water, all day long, every single day, for months straight.

A night of drinking never makes me feel well the next morning. I'm dried out and hungover. I'm usually not hungry for the first half of the day so I miss out on calories. It's easy for me to lose weight. Alcohol also hinders protein synthesis.

Plenty of my friends smoke cannabis, so I usually partake in that if I'm at home. Now that I'm in shape, and a known health nut around my friend, the peer pressure to drink has evaporated. There's nothing wrong with a man or woman focused on their heath goals, as long as they're happy doing so. I never complain in front of friends that I wish I could drink, because I don't.

However, sometimes I do drink a lot. Like on my birthday in June, for example. I avoid beer, because that bothers my stomach the worst. I think it's the yeast so trying other beers fermented with different ingredients may be worthwhile for you if you're into beer. Light vodka coolers or even ciders are probably the best. If the options are too sugary (personal preference), I drink vodka waters. Gin isn't bad either.

If I decide to not drink, but I'm at a nightclub where I'll be socializing with new people or I have a friend that is determined I loosen up by having a drink, it's handy to have a drink in my hand. What do I do?

My friend Don recommended me to drink tonic water with a lime. If you point to the bartender that you want it in a regular glass like the alcohol, they usually will. Sometimes they like to put non-alcoholic drinks in different glasses but be sure to opt out of that, but you'll be treated by bouncers and staff like that is alcoholic, so be mindful of it. Tonic water with a lime tastes great and it looks like alcohol. No one will question you on it.

Even when my liver is in great shape, my inflammation is under control and I know I could get away with a drink or two, I often don't. If you have a hard time quitting alcohol, you could consider the benefits outside of your health. There are many stoic readings available to cover this topic.

With alcohol, similar to drugs, you're escaping reality. Whether, you're in mental pain or physical pain, there's like better and healthier ways to fix this pain. If you're like me, you probably have goals to accomplish. You should be renovating your home or doing meal prep (which we will discuss) or studying for your next exam to promote you in your career.

Everyone has a mission they can focus on to keep them busy. My mission right now is to publish this book, which will be my second book. These are some of the things that have helped me minimize alcohol consumption, and I hope they help you.

Whether you drink alcohol or not, water is extremely important. Alcohol dries you out. When athletes want to lower themselves a few more ounces to make a competition weight, mainly professional bodybuilders, some will drink a glass of wine backstage to make their target weight.

So, how much water should you drink? 70% of the body is water, so a lot. I'm an adult male and when I'm in my rhythm I drink about a gallon a day. If you're a small female, you probably only need half a gallon a day. That's about two liters.

My friend Abbey who's a registered dietician said the best way to tell whether you're drinking enough water is by the color of your urine. Aim to keep it clear. If it's yellow, you aren't drinking enough. If it's red, see a doctor or something. She didn't say that last part – I added that in.

Measuring your water intake isn't the only thing you should be measuring. You will have to start measuring your food at some point, at least until you get good at eyeballing portion sizes. Each person, based on their goal, should aim for a specific ratio of macronutrients, that is, protein, carbohydrates and fats.

Proteins are made of amino acids. There are 20 different amino acids in the human body. 9 of these amino acids are essential meaning you must consume them from food. The others your body can make on its own.

A normal person will consume 0.3 to 0.4 grams of protein for every pound of bodyweight. Someone looking to build muscle, like myself, should eat around 0.8 to 1.2 grams of protein for every pound of bodyweight. I eat closer to 1.2 grams per pound of bodyweight.

Protein is the primary macronutrient in my diet. It's essential for recovery. Often times I found myself abnormally sore, I wasn't eating enough protein.

My favorite protein sources are chicken, wild salmon and egg whites. Red meat is fine if you can digest it. I choose egg whites over regular eggs because I eat them so often and can't be bothered cooking constantly all day. Egg whites in the carton come pasteurized and ready to drink uncooked. If I'm cooking eggs, I'll eat regular eggs rather than cook with egg whites. If I'm drinking or blending them, I'll use egg whites. Each gram of protein contains 4 calories.

Carbohydrates are another macronutrient. They provide energy for the body. Although some will argue, calories as a whole are used for the body's that is true. The body generally sources its energy from carbs consumed and existing body fat. It rarely uses calories from protein, for example, for energy.

There are two types of carbs, simple and complex. Simple carbs give you instant energy. These come from things like fruit or candy. Complex carbs come from starches like potatoes, rice, pasta and grains. These give you long lasting energy throughout the day. Like protein, carbohydrates also contain 4 calories per gram.

The last macronutrient is fatty acids. Fats are also essential in our diet. A big misconception is people think the fats listed are what contributes to body fat, which is not true. More on this later.

Fats are generally one of two different categories, either unsaturated or saturated. While there are exceptions, unsaturated fats are generally considered healthier than saturated fats. Given this book is for beginners, a registered dietician would be able to find exceptions to some of these points, but sometimes simplicity can make learning easier.

Examples of sources of healthy fats include olive oil, avocados, salmon, and nuts. Examples of sources of unhealthy fats include bacon, butter and fried foods.

The word *healthy* is often misunderstood. In this instance, healthy is based on the overall benefits or disadvantages a food brings to the body. Healthy fats help in many different bodily functions including regulating metabolism, transporting oxygen, lowering cholesterol, and even provide energy when glucose (a form of sugar) is not sufficiently available. Unhealthy fats cause cholesterol to build up, raising your LDL (bad) cholesterol.

The word healthy is also used to talk about foods that are high in micronutrients, like whole wheat bread. Whole wheat bread is also considered healthy because it's a source of complex carbs which don't spike glucose levels. Spiking glucose levels will also depend on the individual and the amount consumed so it's not necessary to bash white bread for being much more unhealthy than whole wheat – it's still in the better half of food in the average person's lunch.

Lastly, eating healthy doesn't imply low calorie – or that you'll lose weight. A healthy breakfast could be a couple pieces of toast with avocado. An unhealthy breakfast would be a couple pieces of toast with Smucker's jam. However, if you're looking to lose weight, Smucker's is technically a fine option to fit that goal because it's lower in calories than avocado. So, you can eat healthy and still gain weight – something many beginners don't understand. Fats as a whole are very calorically dense, so while it's important to consume healthy fats, eating too many will easily cause weight gain as each gram of fat contains 9 calories.

Now that we know the basics of each macronutrient and why we consume them (I'm weird and actually think about what my food does for me as I eat it), we need to understand how much we should eat based on our goals.

Gaining weight and losing weight generally come down to your overall caloric intake and expenditure, with the exception of water weight gained by corticosteroids like prednisone. Before going further, I should stop to explain that when you take prednisone, you won't keep all of the gained weight when you stop treatment. Keep your water intake high and sodium intake low then you'll drop that water shortly after you stop prednisone. Prednisone also causes muscle wasting so you'll actually lose muscle when on the drug. Unintentional weight gain from prednisone is only a small part of the journey with IBD.

When not on corticosteroids, weight changes are easily explained by your TDEE. Your body consumes a certain number of calories as maintenance which is called your Total Daily Energy Expenditure (TDEE). Your TDEE depends on many factors such as age, sex, weight, height and activity level. It's incredibly difficult to calculate your TDEE and impossible to pinpoint because there are so many factors but there are multiple calculators online you can use to estimate it.

Once you have an estimated TDEE, you will eat based on your goals. One calculator told me my TDEE is 2809 calories. So, to gain weight, I need to eat in a surplus of 500, and to lose weight, I need to eat in a deficit of 500 calories. Let me write this out using the example of weight gain.

- 2800 calories as maintenance
- +500 calories to gain weight
- +100 calories to account for miscalculations
- +200 calories to account for malabsorption from IBD
- +300 calories to account for extended exercise

The total is about 3900 calories, which is what I am to hit on a daily basis every day. I currently see results with this, and I can tell you, if I only hit 3300 calories per day, I won't gain weight. If I didn't see results, I'd bump the total by 200 calories and test it again for 14 days straight. If you miss a day then start your 14 days over.

It's not only hard to calculate your maintenance but it's incredibly difficult to calculate your malabsorption. Your malabsorption can also change. You only use these estimations to get started, then you track what you eat, record results then make adjustments each week. You may even absorb some foods better or worse than others. Meaning 3900 calories isn't always 3900 calories. Confusing right?

Now let's assume years down the road, I'm around 220 pounds and I want to shred the bodyfat to expose the lean muscular beach body under it, or on the other hand, some people with Crohn's and ulcerative colitis have gained too much weight, usually from living lethargic lives due to joint problems and whatnot, and they want to lose the weight. If the weight gained is water weight (almost always less than 10 pounds), you can shred that by sitting in a bathtub for an hour. You should also cut salt and drink plenty of water (2-4 liters per day). High intensity cardio can help you sweat water weight fairly fast. As for supplements, dandelion root and potassium can help lower water retention.

However, assuming the weight gained is not water weight, calculations may go something like this:

- 2800 calories as maintenance
- -500 calories to lose weight
- -100 calories to account for miscalculations
- +200 calories to account for malabsorption from IBD
- +300 calories to account for extended exercise

This totals 2700 calories. Notice because of malabsorption from IBD, I can still eat an extra 200 calories. If I'm trying to shave bodyfat, I don't have to eat those extra 200 calories, it's just I might feel tired and sluggish if I don't. If you can deal with that feeling, all the power to you, because you'll lose weight faster. However, make sure it's sustainable, if you crash and pig out for a weekend, or even a day, your results will disappear quick. Try to stick to realistic goals that you can happily stick to permanently. Picture your diet as a permanent lifestyle change – not a 90-day challenge like the crap they push in magazines and in commercials.

I also added 300 calories to account for extended exercise in both calculations because I seem to train harder than what most of these calculators estimate and I'll be teaching you how to train hard in part IV.

When gaining weight using the first set of calculations, I'll be gaining body fat and muscle usually at the same time. This is called *bulking*. If you're able to track calories carefully and eat in a 300-400 calorie surplus, you can do what's called *lean bulking*, where you only add muscle (for the most part). However, most people bulk by adding muscle and body fat. Once they get to a heavier weight, they *cut*, which means they adjust their diet to lose weight, which with proper training and a high protein diet, you'll maintain most of your muscle and shed the body fat.

It's important to note that although we are tracking calories on daily basis, what matters is the weekly intake. If I'm trying to eat 3900 calories a day to gain weight, and I hit it on the first day, but I'm too full the next morning, or sick of eating the next day and I only hit 2500 calories, that entire surplus the day before goes to waste. If the goal is 3900 calories per day, I must hit 27300 calories per week.

You don't have to track calories forever. Maybe 6 months. Once you do it for 6 months straight, you should be 100x better at eyeballing calories than you are now. This takes practice and the far majority of people cannot do this. Put the time in now to learn, so you don't have to worry about it later when you're not hitting your goals.

Panasonic has a prototype machine called CaloRieco that scans calories on a plate. In the future I'm hoping devices like that come to market.

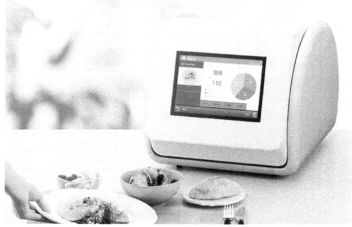

Source: Panasonic.com

The best way to get used to portion sizes and make eating on track easier, is by meal prepping. Once a week, usually on Sunday, you plan out your meals, cook them and put them in the fridge and freezer. There are special containers you can buy and plenty of recipes online you can follow. Usually I leave 3 days' worth of meal prep in the fridge and place the remainder in my freezer, pulling it out the day before and putting it in my fridge to thaw.

I often make shredded chicken by boiling it or using a sous vide. You'll notice shredded chicken reheats in the microwave better than a whole chicken breast. Also, to keep the chicken from getting dry and to add extra calories, you can put some avocado oil (tasteless unlike olive oil) on the chicken before microwaving and cover it with a paper towel. This makes the chicken much less dry than if you were to not.

With my chicken, I choose either rice or sweet potatoes. I really love sweet potatoes because they taste great without anything added. They have the same macronutrients as regular potatoes, but have a few more vitamins and minerals, and taste much better plain. To have a balanced healthy diet, you should also include plenty of your favorite greens with every meal, although they don't help directly with weight gain. They can help by filling you up to make weight loss easier, but they also add all sorts of micronutrients, which we all need.

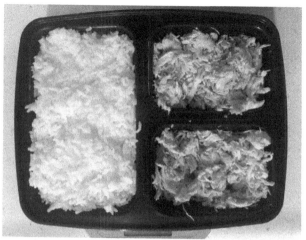
A meal prepped container of white rice and shredded chicken

If you're not getting vitamins and minerals (micronutrients) from food, you should be taking vitamin supplements. Even if you are eating a wide variety of healthy food, it can be a good idea to take supplements.

Iron is normally given via intravenous to IBD patients, as I was, but often a good doctor will put you on a good oral iron supplement after the infusion. Oral is usually used for maintenance, when your values have recovered. Beware as most over the counter iron supplements are difficult to digest, so you must choose carefully. Heme iron is the type of iron extracted from animals, which makes it easier to absorb. A popular brand name is Proferrin, but since it's generally more expensive than the generic, I go with whatever heme iron the pharmacist recommends.

Folic acid (vitamin B9) and Vitamin D3 were the next supplements my doctor told me to take. I won't give you a boring profile of them because they are readily available online. Since people often ask me for my list of supplements to help with weight gain, I should mention I don't attribute my weight gain to any of these listed supplements, they're just what my doctor told me to take. They both have their own set of functions.

The first supplement I take that isn't instructed by my doctor is a comprehensive multi-vitamin. I am not talking about your regular multi-vitamin with a dozen or two vitamins. I'm talking about a vitamin like Optimum Nutrition Opti-Men which contains dozens upon dozens of micronutrients and consequently, they're more expensive than your normal multivitamin.

Micronutrients like Zinc help with natural testosterone levels, which is the hormone that helps build and maintain lean muscle mass, in both men and women. Ladies, do not worry, taking Zinc is not going to lower your voice and grow you a moustache, these are very minor increases in natural levels, which are harmless.

In addition to Zinc, a good multi-vitamin will include Vitamin K which helps with appetite, folic acid if you don't plan on buying that separately, amino acids in case your diet on any given day is lacking protein, and many others which I will not list. These are some basics you can look for if you look at other brands.

I occasionally take protein powders, which are another supplement. Whey protein is the best kind of protein as it has the highest bioavailability, which means it absorbs best. The next best would be meat-based protein powders like Redcon1 MRE which is used by the World's Strongest Man, Brian Shaw. Pea protein is excellent for vegans, or those who can't have whey and can't afford some of the meat proteins. Most vegan proteins don't mix as well as whey protein.

When it comes to whey protein there are a few kinds. Casein is a slow digesting low-grade whey. It's also super cheap. Whey concentrate is mid-grade. Whey isolate is the highest grade of whey protein. It can be filtered to the point of being considered virtually lactose free, carbohydrate free, fat free, and cholesterol free.

This is how I consume whey even when I consider my diet to be dairy free. A high-quality whey isolate has minimal casein or lactose. As I mentioned earlier, it's important to re-test your diet to make sure your past findings are accurate. Which led me to retesting dairy mildly, by adding highly filtered whey protein into my diet. I still don't eat cheese, butter or milk but the benefits of highly filtered whey are hard to fully ignore whereas the benefits of the other dairy products listed are usually just flavor, something I have the willpower to go without. So, I've been taking whey protein lately. It's also much cheaper than drinking raw egg whites.

I used to eat egg white protein powder but later switched it out for raw egg whites. The bioavailability in raw egg whites is not high, but it's easy to drink a lot of them to make up for that. A good source of protein powder is TrueNutrition.com where you can make any blend, from any source, of any flavor, of any intensity, with any added micronutrients… it's pretty amazing. I'm not sponsored by them but should be.

For a popular protein blend like whey, it can be cheaper to buy a pre-made jug from Amazon or similar. My favorite brands of whey are Diesel and Allmax Isoflex. I don't mind Cellucor Isolate and Optimum Nutrition Gold Standard are also decent options in my experience. The list of whey brands are endless. I like something that is considered lactose-free, tastes great and mixes well. Check the ingredient label to make sure that whey isolate is first on the list and not whey concentrate. A good whey will be made of 90% or more isolate.

The last supplement I take is a good pre-workout which I'll add to my water bottle before I go to the gym. Caffeine can sometimes act as a laxative so be careful. I also sometimes take BCAAs, usually just to flavor my water as I don't really need them due to all the protein I eat. These two are often combined into one product, but not always. BCAAs are 3 amino acids, but lately there's been a lot of buzz around EAAs, which include all 9 of the essential amino acids. If you're eating the amount of protein you're supposed to be, from meat sources, you won't need BCAAs or EAAs. A pre-workout is nice as it can give you some energy before the gym, but sometimes I'm just naturally so excited to go put on muscle, I don't really need it.

PART IV: TRAINING

Similar to lifestyle changes and diet, exercise alone also cannot heal Crohn's disease. Exercise is proven to improve both physiological and psychological health in Crohn's disease patients. Additionally, diminished qualities normally found in Crohn's disease patients such as bone mineral density, quality of life, body mass index and muscle mass also show improvement.[26]

Throughout the book, I tend to refer to exercise as *training* or *lifting* because exercise as a whole can refer to a multitude of things. Specifically, I believe weight training is one of the most effective ways to gain strength and increase confidence along with overall quality of life. While yoga and Pilates are also exercise, they aren't the most effective way of getting to a healthy body. There are only upsides if you'd still like to add them in.

Training in the gym only takes 3 sessions per week, and about 45 minutes per session. The more sessions you do, generally the

---

[26] Ng, Victor et al. "Exercise and Crohn's disease: speculations on potential benefits." Canadian journal of gastroenterology = Journal canadien de gastroenterologie vol. 20,10 (2006): 657-60. doi:10.1155/2006/462495

better the results, but I'd say the majority of results can be obtained at 3-4 sessions per week – and you don't need to spend hours there. You could even pack a workout into an intense 30-40 minutes before or after work, but I usually aim for an hour, give or take.

Training earlier in the day is my preference. With IBD, chronic fatigue is quite common, so I prioritize my important things earlier in the day, like my training. Fatigue is probably the biggest side effect I have from the disease, so you'll learn to plan a lifestyle around the lethargy that introduces. You could also nap later in the day and then train when you wake up. Remember, sleep is growth so don't hesitate.

Going to the gym, if you've never been a fan, is not as intimidating as most are led to believe. If you stay humble and focus on your lifts, and your form, no one will bother you. Bring headphones to listen to music, as you may get sick of the music your gym plays. Sometimes I wear a hoodie, which signifies to others in a friendly way, I'm focused on myself and do not want to be disturbed. I like to be left alone. Feel free to wear the same.

People have a perception of gym goers, in that they workout to look good for the opposite sex, and that is true, much of the opposite sex is attracted to fit, healthy people, but it shouldn't be your core motivation. If you're not working out for yourself and only yourself, you're going to give up. Work out because it's healthy. It makes you strong. It makes you sleep better. You build a routine, confidence, ambition... you learn discipline. You learn to stick to the plan and to track progress. You learn to break through excuses and plateaus. If you're a guy, it builds natural testosterone. If you have a disease like Crohn's, it can make you live a longer, healthier, happier life.

So, once you've decided to make the leap, it's time to find a gym. I live in a small town, so my options are limited but I still have to use a few factors when considering.

The first factor is what equipment is available and what equipment you need. You need a gym with barbells and a squat rack. You need a gym with dumbbells that go from 5 pounds up to 100 pounds. You don't need a gym with 75 treadmills, unless you're trying to lose weight, but even then, you only need one that's available. Don't let excess amounts of cardio equipment distract you in your decision. You don't care about their Zumba classes or their squash courts. You are there to lift heavy weights.

Next, consider their hours, when are they open? Are they open 7 days a week? Most serious gyms are. Are they open before work, and after work? Are they open after your children go to bed?

Next, consider the distance and the commute. If you're driving, GPS the gyms from your house, and consider the difference. A gym that is 5 minutes away, will be a lot more convenient when you're driving there several times a week than one that's 15 minutes away. Don't choose the one that is 15 minutes away because your friend goes there.

Lastly, if you have limited options, a bigger gym is usually a better gym. More equipment, more equipment options.

Sometimes at a new gym, you'll get a free session with a trainer, who will teach you some of the equipment to get started. YouTube is great for learning new routines and exercises to perfect your form, and your workout strategy. However, I can firmly say I wouldn't be where I am if it wasn't for my trainers. They helped me a lot. They show you what it means to train with intensity. I don't train with trainers often anymore, mainly because my hometown lacks qualified trainers, but when I visit my parents in Fort Myers, I love to train with a successful trainer.

They can help you develop a training routine, give you feedback on your meal plan, answer any questions, keep things exciting, help you push through every last possible rep, making sure you get the most out of your workout. They can help you feel comfortable in the gym, introduce you to familiar faces in the gym, and really make it feel like home.

I found both my trainers through Instagram. You can also ask your gym's front desk for trainer recommendations. There will probably be some trainers there with clients when you stop in for the first time. I liked picking my trainers on Instagram before my first day at the new gym, because I was able to critique them based on their physique and have them meet me there the day I joined. If they look like exaggerated versions of what I want to look like, then I was interested. I didn't want a trainer that was skinny or fat. If they are under the age of 50, they should be in great shape. Older, semi-retired trainers, who sit on a pile of knowledge from decades of professional sports experience, are the only exception but they have trophies and vintage photos to show you what they can obtain with their knowledge.

I do want to suggest not hiring a trainer that works out of a private studio. A trainer has many benefits and you're not getting many of them if you're in a studio. Generally, you're only allowed to workout at the studio if you're with your trainer. If you have a trainer for every workout, this gets expensive quick and it doesn't let up because going to the gym isn't a temporary fix but a permanent lifestyle change.

A trainer helps build confidence in the gym so you're more inclined to go more frequently. They show you different equipment and how to properly use it. You'll learn how to work out on your own by the 4th or 5th session. I can vividly remember going through that transition to my first solo gym visit in November of 2018. Like anything else in life, by obtaining an understanding of what you're doing, you will gain confidence.

Whether you use a trainer or not, you will decide on a training split. This partly depends on how many days per week you plan to train and what your overall goals are. For example, someone who trains to look good will often have a program that has days which focus on smaller muscle groups like arms and shoulders for example, whereas someone training to be strong will often not, and they'll focus on bigger muscle groups, like legs, chest and back.

The three main goals you can choose from are:

- Training to be strong (power)
- Training to look strong (muscle mass)
- Training for endurance (cardiovascular health)

Training to be strong means focusing on explosive strength. While generally muscle equates to strength, it's not always true. A 220-pound powerlifter is much stronger than a 220-pound bodybuilder. To build strength, it's best to focus on heavy weight. Given you're lifting near your max, your sets will be in low rep ranges (<6). You'll have less than 10 sets per session and have large rest times between sets (2-10 minutes).

Training to look strong means focusing on growing the muscle to the maximum size through hypertrophy. This is great for boosting confidence through appearance and is the quickest way to put on muscle. Athletes training for hypertrophy often work in the 8-12 rep range for many of their sets. They frequently have 14-18 sets per workout and often rest 30-60 seconds between sets.

Training for endurance also includes training for longevity and overall health. This includes HIIT training programs and other training styles that involves a large number of reps. This is the only training style I don't participate much in as it's generally best for those looking to lose weight by burning the most calories. All styles can be used to gain/lose weight based on food intake, but some are more optimal than others for certain goals. Training for endurance means lots of sets, lots of reps and very little rest time. The weight used is also the lowest of all training styles.

It's important to note the rep ranges for each goal are not always within those ranges. A powerlifter may squat sets of 3 reps then after finishing their squats, do a few isolations with machines for 12 reps. A bodybuilder may do sets of 12 reps then on their last set do a burn out AMRAP (as many reps as possible) set where they go for 20+ reps at a light weight to finish the day.

The most basic, 3-day routine is a full body routine. Monday, Wednesday and Friday you train compound movements, which are movements that use many different muscles like the squat, bench press, deadlift, pull up, dip, row and military press. The other days, you rest. This routine will get you results but do not fall to 1 or 2 days per week or you may be stuck in a maintenance routine with little to no growth.

If you want to gain strength, you can follow a powerlifting program. Each program is different and there are many online. When I was growing my deadlift, I switched to a powerlifting program and it went something like this.

Day	Activity
1	Squat and bench
2	Rest
3	Deadlift
4	Rest

The benefit with a program like this is you're able to hit all 3 major compound movements nearly twice per week. If you are finding you can't recover enough from squat for your deadlift day or vice versa, you could do a variation like this.

Day	Activity
1	Squat (leg day)
2	Bench (push day)
3	Rest
4	Deadlift (pull day)
5	Bench (push day)
6	Rest

A program like that allows you to bench twice a week and still give you two days of recovery between, which is ideal for most guys looking to focus on upper body strength.

When training for strength, you focus on lifting heavy in the 2-5 rep range. 5x5 is common. That's 5 sets of 5 repetitions. Also, with powerlifting, your rest time between sets is 2-5 minutes because the sets are very exhausting and heavy. You will likely do 2 exercises like flat bench and incline bench, meaning a full workout would consist of only 10 sets, or if you do 4x4 for 2 exercises, only 8 sets. Your program may even have you do 3x3 one week. This type of program will make you stronger.

Over the years I've hired some of the strongest men in the world with deadlifts in excess of 800 and even 1000 pounds to make me programs. I'm going to share two of these programs as I believe if you can read them, analyze them and understand them, it will dramatically help you in your strategies.

The first program is a program designed for me by 308-pound Chris Wiest. It's an 8-week program designed to increase my deadlift. The program was based on my max at the time of 340 pounds.

Week 1	Weight	Sets	Reps	Total Reps
Deadlift	280	2	5	10
Back Raises	X	3	10	30
DB SLDL	X	3	10	30
Leg Extensions	X	3	10	30
Lat Pull Downs/ DB Rows	X	4	10	80

Week 2	Weight	Sets	Reps	Total Reps
Deadlift	295	1	4	4
Back Raises	X	3	10	30
DB SLDL	X	3	10	30
Leg Extensions	X	3	10	30
Lat Pull Downs/ DB Rows	X	4	10	80

Week 3	Weight	Sets	Reps	Total Reps
Deadlift	305	4	2	8
Back Raises	X	3	10	30
DB SLDL	X	3	10	30
Leg Extensions	X	3	10	30
Lat Pull Downs/ DB Rows	X	4	10	40

Week 4	Weight	Sets	Reps	Total Reps
Deadlift	255	3	3	9
Back Raises	X	3	10	30

DB SLDL	X	3	10	30
Leg Extensions	X	3	10	30
Lat Pull Downs/ DB Rows	X	4	10	40

Week 5	Weight	Sets	Reps	Total Reps
Deadlift	315	4	1	4
Back Raises	X	3	10	30
DB SLDL	X	3	10	30
Leg Extensions	X	3	10	30
Lat Pull Downs/ DB Rows	X	4	10	40

Week 6	Weight	Sets	Reps	Total Reps
Deadlift	325	2	1	2
Back Raises	X	3	10	30
DB SLDL	X	3	10	30
Leg Extensions	X	3	10	30
Lat Pull Downs/ DB Rows	X	4	10	40

Week 7: Deload 55-60% 3x3
Week 8: Go for a personal record!

You can reverse engineer this program by looking at it in percentages. For example, week 1 is 2x5 at 82% of my max. The next program is another deadlift program. This program was also made for me by another elite-level powerlifter.

Week 1 Workout 1
Deadlift 85% x 1 x 3 sets

Week 1 Workout 2
Paused Deadlift 80% x 1 x 3 sets

Week 2 Workout 1
Deadlift 90% x 1
Deadlift 85% x 1 x 2

Week 2 Workout 2
Deficit Deadlift 85% x1
Deficit Deadlift 80% x1 x 2

Week 3 Workout 1
Deadlift 95% x 1
Deadlift 90% x 1
Deficit Deadlift 75% x 1

Week 3 Workout 2
Deficit Deadlift 90% x 1
Deficit Deadlift 85% x 1 x 2

Week 4 Workout 1
Deadlift 95% x 1
Deadlift 90% x 1 x 2
Paused Deadlift 87.5% x 1 x 2

Week 4 Workout 2
Paused Deadlift 95% x 1
Paused Deadlift 90% x 1 x 2

Week 5 Workout 1
Deadlift 90% x 1 x 3

Week 5 Workout 2
Deadlift 100% x 1
Deficit Deadlift 90% x 1 x 2

Week 6 Workout 1
Deficit Deadlift 92.5% x 1
Paused Deficit Deadlift 85% x 1 x 2

Week 6 Workout 2
Deadlift 92.5% x 1 x 3

Week 7 Workout 1
Deadlift 97.5% x 1
Deficit Deadlift 92.5% x 1
Paused Deficit 85% x 1

Week 7 Workout 2
Deficit Deadlift 95% x 1
Deficit Deadlift 90% x 1 x 2

Week 8 Workout 1
Deadlift 92.5% x 1 x 3

Week 8 Workout 2
Deadlift 102.5% x 1

These programs may not be an asset to you as a beginner, but once you turn novice and hit your first plateau, they can help you break through. In the beginning, you will be advancing weights fairly consistently, so a program won't do much good until your growth slows - maybe 6-12 months in.

The second method of training is bodybuilding. Bodybuilding is the art involved in making the body look good. In bodybuilding, you focus on training specific muscles, rather than training movements like a powerlifter would. Both strategies build muscle, but powerlifters are stronger and explosive, and bodybuilders look better, generally.

Earlier we talked about a beginner program that involves a full body workout, 3 times per week. As a bodybuilder, you'll want to train more frequently. If you are able to train 4-5 days per week, you can consider an upper/lower split. Quite simply, one day you focus on upper body movements and the next you focus on lower body movements. You take a rest day if needed (you should be sore) and you repeat. You could do this twice per week to train 4 days per week, with rest days on Wednesday, Saturday and Sunday.

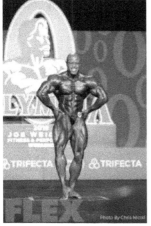

Another split you can consider is sometimes nicknamed the *bro split*, which is what I did for a while, and many bodybuilders do too. It's a bodybuilding program as it breaks the body down into smaller groups and focuses on targeting all muscles at different points in the week. It's not as efficient as others as you are paying time to build smaller muscles like the bicep when you could be training a bigger muscle group which would add mass faster, but I like it as it gives every muscle attention and my trainer, IFBB Pro Lloyd Dollar, put me on this routine. I trust him because he's one of the best in the world. Pictured is him on the Mr. Olympia stage. 1 of 5 Americans on the stage that year in the 212 class.

My routine changes often, but with this kind of split, it goes something like this:

Sun	Mon	Tues	Wed	Thurs	Fri	Sat
Back	Chest	Legs	Rest	Shoulders	Arms	Rest

On chest day I'll also hit triceps and on my back day I'll also hit biceps and forearms. This means my full arm gets a workout twice a week.

This routine ensures I'm able to isolate all muscles during the week. So instead of training the body as a whole, I train each part individually, which may sound like the same, but like I said earlier, it will get more focus on arms, shoulders and other smaller muscles, which are mainly for aesthetics.

The last routine I want to recommend is a 6-day routine and it's called push-pull-legs or PPL. You can do this twice per week, with a rest day at the end. It allows you to train legs (leg day) and back (pull day) twice per week, given they are two of the biggest muscle groups in the body. A program like this is balanced for strength and muscle gain because you're hitting the big muscle groups but also hitting them frequently. It's not optimal for strength if that's your single goal as you won't be able to train super hard as you won't be fully recovered, and you'll have a hard time fueling up on food when working out so much and constantly burning calories. Classic Physique Olympia champion and fellow Canadian Chris Bumstead recently mentioned in a YouTube video that he made the transition to a PPL program.

If you're doing a bodybuilding routine, each day you'll choose anywhere between 3 to 6 different exercises to do, and generally I aim for 16-20 sets per workout. More sets is not always better as you'll start burning too many calories. It's also a tell-tale sign that you aren't training hard enough as you're still alive after 20 sets. All you want to do is exhaust the muscle by heavy, intense lifting for a shorter period of time. I like to incorporate both compounds and isolations in my routine.

Each day you'll prioritize your most important (usually compound) lifts at the start of your routine. On leg day, this would be squats. On back day, this would be deadlifts. On chest day, this would be bench press and/or dips. On shoulder day, this would be military press. After these powerful exercises, you switch to isolations and start targeting specific accessory muscles. On shoulder day, you break down the shoulder into the 3 heads - the anterior (front delt), medial (side delt) and posterior (rear delt). This makes 4 movements for the day – the compound movement to start followed by isolation movements for each head. 4 movements with 4 sets each brings you to 16 sets which is a great session.

I'm not going to break down the programs and workouts much deeper as the bodybuilding community on YouTube is quite comprehensive on some of this information. Go on YouTube and type in "upper lower split" for example, and you'll get a full routine to try. You can also find some movements and tutorials on my Conquer Crohn's YouTube channel as well. Browse YouTube to visually see the movements and programs demonstrated in a gym.

This brings me to my next point. Before each session, you should have a plan in your head of the exercises you plan to do that day. You have a rough order of how you'd like to do them, but if a machine is busy, you have no issue doing one before the other unless it's your first lift. It's hard to start the leg day with anything but the squat rack. You could warm up and stretch. You could foam roll for a bit. You could go to the leg extension machine and do some light work to get your quads ready to lift.

You can review proper form in a quick video on YouTube to remind yourself what you're doing so when you get to your station and you're good to go. Sometimes when I'm squatting or deadlifting, I'll notice in the mirror someone staring at me. When I'm done my set, if it's obvious they are a gym goer that knows what they're doing, I'll turn, look them in the eyes and motion thumb up or thumbs down. They'll either give thumbs up if my form was good or they'll walk over and give feedback. It's always nice to get criticism from 3rd person. It's essential for efficient and quick progress when you're not with a trainer. Even the best in the world work with a trainer.

Unlike powerlifting, when bodybuilding, in each lift, you must focus not just on moving the weight, but establishing a mind-muscle connection, which is the conscious and deliberate muscle contraction. So, if you're curling a dumb bell, a beginner would just try to move the dumb bell through the motion. We all know what that looks like, so it's easy to do. However, you should focus on contracting your bicep muscle, like you do when you flex your bicep when you have nothing heavy in your hand. That's a mind-muscle connection. So, contract your bicep when you curl. It can be handy to roll up your sleeve, look in the mirror, whatever is necessary to optimally view the muscle. Your trainer will often poke at the muscle with their finger to check if you're contracting properly and to help you feel where the muscle is that you're contracting. This can be helpful for a muscle you can't see, like an area of your back. If you can see the muscle, like your bicep or chest, often looking at it and focusing on it will be enough. When doing curls, your shoulders and back should not be swinging to help. When doing rows, your back should be doing the work, not your bicep. These are common things you'll be considering when establishing a proper mind-muscle connection.

While it can be easy during your first rep to keep perfect form, this gets harder as the reps progress and the lactic acid within your muscles build up throughout the set. You'll need to carefully plan the perfect number of sets and reps for each exercise. You'll also need to choose the right weight so that by the last repetition, you have zero strength left to do another, even if I was to pay you a million dollars to do 1 more.

In a bodybuilding routine, I generally aim to do around 16-20 sets per workout. If I'm doing lots of exercises, I may do 2 or 3 sets each. If I'm doing few exercises, I'll likely do 4 sets each.

In my compound movements, I'll warm up with a light weight, high reps, and then I'll start my first real set that I count, with a good amount of weight, and do a low amount of reps. I'll add weight after each set. If I can do more than 8 reps, the weight I chose wasn't high enough. By my last set, say of deadlifts, I'm only squeezing out 1 to 3 reps.

Later in my workout, I'm doing isolations, and this is where I sometimes like to crank up the repetitions during isolates. I'll go for 20 or 30 reps during my last set of an isolation exercise, called a burnout set. Sometimes I'll do a superset, which is going from one exercise to another that focuses on another muscle, with no rest in between, going back and forth, and I'll end up doing 60, 70 or 80 reps with no rest.

Biceps, for example, are efficient muscles, so you really have

CONQUER CROHN'S

to hit them hard, and their recovery is quick, so you can hit them many times per week. For a burnout set, say I was curling 25-pound dumb bells for 20 reps (10 each side) for 5 sets. I may throw in a 6th set immediately after the 5th where I drop the 25-pound dumb bells and pick up the 10 or 15s and do as many as I can. This is painful and the growth feels great.

Earlier in my journey, I asked my IFBB trainer whether he likes a routine of high reps with low weight or low reps with high weight his response was "High reps, high weight!" which basically means, you need to train with high intensity. Always be pushing the number of reps you can get, and always be pushing the weight you can do. Don't let risk of injury prevent you from training with intensity. Understand how to safely handle larger weights and continue to push forward. Be sure to get aggressive with your training so you can see results after your first few months. Often if people don't see their beginner results, they lose motivation and eventually stop all together. Remember, you have a low chance of injury if your form is correct and if you work in the 6+ rep range your risk of injury is low. Injury is more common when powerlifters are trying to gain strength in the 1-3 rep range which means they're lifting very heavy. Regardless of your rep range, your goal is to have 0-2 reps left in the tank for the given weight. That's the intensity you want. Near the end of the workout, your final sets should be to failure meaning 0 reps left in the tank. In the words of Greg Doucette, if I theoretically gave you a million dollars for each additional rep at the end of your last set, how many more could you do? It should be zero.

While on the note of training hard, overtraining is also rare. Many people worry about it who shouldn't. If you're overtraining, you'll know because you're at the gym for 3 hours a day, 7 days a week. If that's you, you're probably not home eating enough to fuel all that exercise, so it isn't helping you gain weight anymore. 6 hours in the gym per week (including warmup, foam rolling and whatnot) is often all you'll ever need. That's 6 sessions of 1-hour per week or 3 sessions of 2-hours each.

You can add time in the gym if you're doing cardio and stretching, but cardio is usually not something people do much of when trying to gain weight. However, a touch of cardio is good for everyone to keep your heart happy. Our goal, being underweight with IBD, is to put on muscle mass in the easiest way possible, while sticking to a strict, clean diet. The more cardio you do, the more you will have to eat to counter the calories you've burned. If you just want to do some cardio to stay in good health, 3 times a week you can run a quick mile, hit a bag for a couple of 3-minute rounds, or skip rope at high pace for 3-4 minutes. Otherwise, stay off the treadmills, ellipticals, bikes and rowing machines unless you have a good reason to use them if you goal is to gain weight quickly.

One thought that beginners often have is that they "don't want to get too big" which makes experienced lifters chuckle, because it's hard to get too big. You don't get big by accident. It takes years to do that, and you're well aware of the signs of where you're headed while on your journey.

Those guys you see in magazines who have massive muscles and veins popping out have worked for decades, eating 6 meals a day, in addition to possessing superior genetics to achieve their physiques. They didn't stop at their natural limit. You don't get too big accidentally, so don't even think about that idea at all.

The only way you could get too big was if you got fat, and that's from eating too much. When I say fat, I mean you have a high body fat percentage, not that your bodyweight is high.

I think it's important beginners understand body fat and how it influences a physique. A bodyweight doesn't tell the full story of someone's physique. Body fat percentage in conjunction with height and weight draw the most accurate picture. My body fat percentage last checked was 7.24% which means I'm very lean. It doesn't mean skinny without mapping that body fat calculation to a height and weight. You could be 240 pounds and jacked at 7% bodyfat or 100 pounds and skinny at 7% body fat. A low body fat percentage means you have abs. You can have abs at 120 pounds, and you can have abs at 220 pounds. Let me show you some examples of people at 7% body fat.

CONQUER CROHN'S

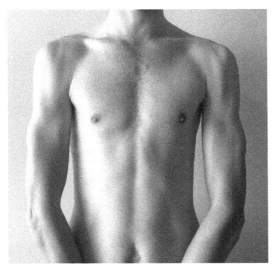

This is me in 2018. ~125 pounds and 7% body fat.

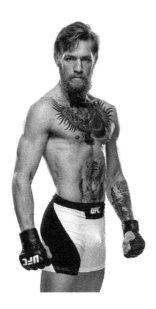

Conor McGregor at ~154 pounds and 7% body fat.

CONQUER CROHN'S

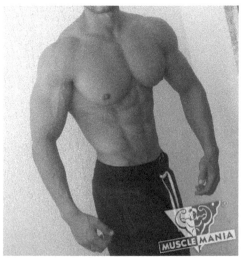

Also 7% body fat but at 210 pounds.

You can see, low body fat doesn't mean skinny or big. It can be either. The amount of muscle they have is not determined by bodyfat percentages. Now that you've seen different weights at the same body fat, I think it's important to look at how different body fats look.

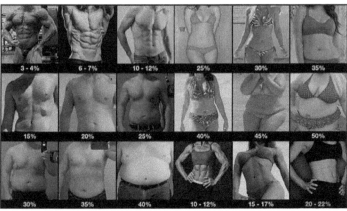

Different body fats for men and women.

72

So, what is "too big" (in terms of muscles) anyways? The average person thinks you're too big if you're high in weight, while maintaining low body fat. If you are missing either of those requirements, you won't look too muscular. If you have a bit of extra body fat, you won't. If you have a lower overall body weight, you won't.

If your goal is to look good, you have to consider, is that with or without a shirt on? A smaller guy at 165 pounds with 10% body fat will look great on the beach, but small with a shirt on. However, the same guy with extra body fat putting him at 178 with 18% body fat will look better with a shirt on, because he fills out the shirt more, without looking chubby.

If you're like me, aim to be around 8-12% body fat, and which bodyweight that corresponds to will depend on your height. As a 6'2 male, I would look good around 190-210 pounds lean. This takes years and can be a daunting task when staring at that number while on a scale that reads 120 pounds, but with proper sleep, nutrition, medication and training, you can get to this point.

I wish you the best of the luck in your journey. My physique has salvaged my self-esteem, boosting my confidence and mental health to uncharted levels. It causes people to look at me and treat me different and has changed my life in unbelievable ways. With my newfound confidence, it's evident I'm not afraid to go after everything and anything I want in life and I wish the same for each one of you. Good luck and Godspeed.

ABOUT THE AUTHOR

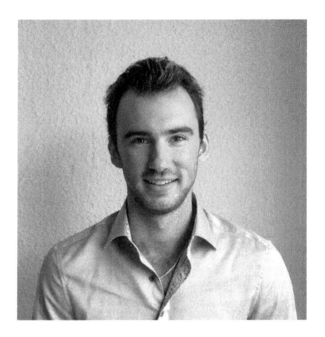

Josh MacDonald is a Canadian author and entrepreneur. He grew up in Turkey Point, Ontario while building a profitable software company throughout high school. While attending the University of Toronto for computer science, he built and sold the software company SerpClix from his Toronto bachelor pad. After the acquisition and graduation, he focused on his disease, and determined to gain weight and sculpt a healthy physique, has now gained over 50 pounds since diagnosis.

Media inquiries: josh@joshmacdonald.net

CONQUER CROHN'S

BEFORE

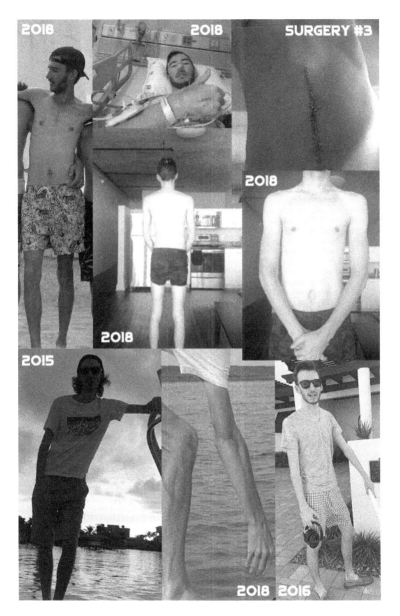

CONQUER CROHN'S

AFTER

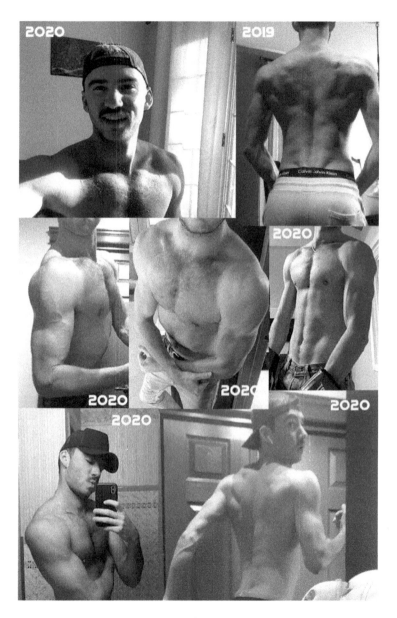

CONQUER CROHN'S

Milton Keynes UK
Ingram Content Group UK Ltd.
UKHW041519280724
1059UKWH00018B/139